Free Your Voice: Heal Your Thyroid

REVERSE THYROID DISEASE NATURALLY

ROSANNE LINDSAY, ND, MA

Cover design by Karen Nelson and onceandfuture
Edit by Patricia Mansi
Book design by onceandfuture and Anne Temple
Copy Edit by Darlene Oakey

ISBN/SKU: 9780692108703
ISBN Complete: 978-0-692-10870-3

Library of Congress Control Number: 2018907663

Lindsay Publishing
http://www.natureofhealing.org

For you, the healer…
What I've learned about healing thyroid disease
Comes through my own experience,
Using body-mind-spirit medicine.
Within these pages I move my innovation
Forward through you.
Together we send healing ripples out
To affect all life.

Contents

ACKNOWLEDGMENTS

Healing doesn't happen in a void, and so I wish to express my appreciation and love to those who've walked this journey with me in one way or another.

Deep love goes to my family; my children who embody the spirit of adventure, reminding me that healing is about freedom; and my parents for their example of unconditional love and courage in taking on the role of raising me.

To my cherished friends, and the many healers who guided me, and those who have encouraged and nudged me to open and express my gifts so they can be shared, thank you for showing up and doing your own important work. You all know who you are and I love you.

Thank you to my editor, Patricia Manzi, for your care and wisdom of phrasing, comical notes, and attention to detail in transforming the words from my manuscript into a book the reader can appreciate. And also to the talented Karen Nelson, friend and graphic artist extraordinaire, for your artistic eye in creating the book cover design.

For your words of support, thank you Dr. David Brownstein, iodine doctor, author, and compassionate healer. You led me, and so many others, to understand the healing power of iodine in the reversal of thyroid disease, through your many books, especially *Iodine, Why You Need It, Why You Can't Live Without It.*

Thank you, Scott Tips for your review and comments. As President and General Counsel for the National Health Federation, your work on food and drug laws helps protect people's freedom to choose how to heal themselves.

Myron Eshowsky, gifted shaman, author, and teacher, thank you for your example in navigating the spirit world, for your words of support for this book, and for the gift of your own book, *Peace with Cancer.*

Note to the Reader

My healing journey began with a diagnosis of Profound Hypothyroidism. As someone who questions everything, I first went looking for answers in books and scientific journals to understand my condition. As I gathered the evidence my mind required, no amount of research prepared me for what spirit had arranged.

This book furthers the discussion of body-mind-spirit medicine begun in my first book, *The Nature of Healing, Heal the Body, Heal the Planet*. While each chapter builds upon the last, there is no clear beginning or end. As art imitates life, this book evolves without a roadmap, so feel free to skip around in any order and go where spirit leads you. In other words, enjoy the ride. The destination matters not.

In sharing my story of disease reversal, my intention is to change the narrative and present options to the mindset of *living with disease* so you can make informed choices and heal yourself. Disease is a departure from health. Yet, if we observe Natural Law and honor the body's self-regenerating power, disease can be reversed and health restored.

The choices presented herein are not all that exist. No claims for usage, dosage, diagnosis, prescription, treatment, or cure are intended. Nothing in these pages is meant to replace standard therapies or to be used to delay seeking standard treatment. Such decisions should be made between a client and his or her holistic health provider or health team.

It is important to know that, as each person is an original, there are different ways of being, and more than one way to heal. That said, if you have a medical condition, seek the advice of a medical doctor. And, as always, do your own research.

Also by Rosanne Lindsay:

The Nature of Healing, Heal The Body, Heal The Planet

For information on courses, blogs, videos, and articles
by Rosanne Lindsay, visit www.natureofhealing.org

Introduction

From Victimhood
to Freedom

The health of the Earth is embodied in the health of her people. As we come to realize that humanity is connected at the level of our health, national borders and political parties become irrelevant. Today, the silent epidemic of thyroid disease is not only a universal phenomenon but also a reflection of how the people have lost their collective voice. Silence and powerlessness go hand in hand. When we suppress our ability to speak truth, we manifest it in the physical.

The thyroid is a butterfly-shaped gland, both physical and metaphysical in nature. It is located at the base of the throat, and also housed in the fifth energy center...the throat chakra...of the energy body. The physical thyroid requires iodine to manage energy for every cell in the body, as well as to regulate heart function. The metaphysical thyroid governs communication powers of all types, verbal and bodily, as well as balances self-expression and creative expression.

Women are ten times more likely than men to be diagnosed

with thyroid disease, the majority being underactive thyroid disease, or hypothyroidism. Of those with a thyroid condition, eighty percent are autoimmune.[1][2]

Autoimmunity exists when the body decides that healthy cells are foreign invaders and mounts an attack against itself. In this unfortunate case of "friendly fire," our bodies become reluctant victims of our environment and of our choices—from the foods we eat to the thoughts we think.

The attack of Self defines the Age of Victimhood. In this book, we will explore the idea that we are the cause of our disease. Our condition did not manifest overnight. We did not see it coming to prepare for it. The transformation began as a slow boil as we dissolved our connection to Nature over time.

Outside of Nature, our world is one of duality—self vs. other. A dualistic dynamic creates isolation, conflict, opposition, and imbalance. An imbalance of the throat chakra can result in the loss of voice or hoarseness, and the fear of being exposed. Perhaps women are more susceptible to autoimmune disease if they grow up in a patriarchal society, conditioned to favor others over themselves. From the workplace to the home front, women have learned to give without receiving and to let others speak for them. If not careful, they drain their energy without replenishing it, not realizing the quality of energy is essential to the quality of life.

In his classic *Inquiries Into Human Faculty*, English Victorian author Francis Galton declared energy to be the measure of fullness of life, vitality, and sensitivity. In Galton's world of 1833, it was well established that the amount of energy of each individual is a function of the thyroid. The greater the thyroid function, the more energetic, quick thinking, and sensitive the individual. The lower the thyroid function, the less energetic, slow thinking, and less sensitive. Sensitivity is a function of the connection between endocrine and nervous systems. Underlying the flow of energy is the amount of activated iodine in the body.[3]

Two hundred years ago, the practice of medicine embraced a holistic view of the individual as part of Nature. Today, modern medicine takes a reductionist view. Holistic medicine is an art, while modern medicine is a science. Holism sees mind and body as one, whereas modern medicine separates mind and body into systems. Holism includes the spirit, where the whole is more than the sum of its parts. Modern medicine says the body is a machine broken down into biological, chemical, and physical components. Holism focuses on caring to guide the patient to heal himself, deferring to the wisdom of the body, or body consciousness. Modern medicine places the keys to the patient's body into the doctor's hands.

When disease is the focus of medicine, it creates a self-fulfilling prophecy: If people believe they are powerless, they behave in a powerless way. All autoimmune disease, whether hypothyroidism, autism, or Alzheimer's, are epidemics of imbalance in body, mind, soul, and spirit.

Physically, we are nutritionally out of balance because of toxins in our food, air, water, and medications. Instead of removing the chemicals and metals to reverse the damage, we standardize it. We overmedicate, open more Assisted Living Centers, and market an autistic doll as "the new normal."

It is a myth that Americans live longer today. Studies confirm our diseased state:

> LIVING SICK AND DYING YOUNG—In 2008, America ranked 47th in the world for life expectancy.[4]
>
> According to the Starfield Report in the 2000 Journal Of the American Medical Association, allopathic medicine is the third leading cause of death, responsible for 225,000 total deaths per year by iatrogenic (medically-induced) causes, including 2038 deaths per week from prescription drugs alone.[5]
>
> A 2013 report in the *Journal of Patient Safety*[6] showed

preventable medical errors persist as the No. 3 killer in the U.S. claiming the lives of some 400,000 people, third only to heart disease and cancer,[7] which are plausible byproducts of allopathic medicine.

The 2013 U.S. Health in International Perspective reported Americans spend the most on healthcare yet live shorter lives and represent the sickest nation in the world in all age groups.[8]

The 2014 Mirror Mirror On The Wall report by the Commonwealth Fund showed that among eleven industrialized nations, the U.S. underperforms in health outcomes at age sixty, and in infant mortality.[9] A 2014 update put the U.S. as dead last among first world nations in health status.[10]

From a 2016 study, medical errors are the third leading cause of death in America at 251,000 deaths per year. This does not include severe patient injuries from medical error, which is 40 times the death rate, or 10 million. More Americans are dying from the care they receive rather than from the disease.[11]

Sixty percent of Americans are prescribed a prescription drug to compensate for an imbalance. To escape pain, people are told to take synthetic opioids. In 2016, the opioid epidemic took 42,000 American lives, while overdose deaths from all drugs took the lives of 64,000 Americans the same year, an increase of 21 percent over the previous year. According to the Citizens Commission on Human Rights, more than one million American kids younger than six are taking psychiatric drugs. We are a nation under sedation.[12]

We presume clinical trials carried out on drugs are published before they are approved and marketed. We trust what we are told even though we are not told that half of all clinical trials never publish results.[13] We are not told that trials that give a positive result are twice as likely to be published as trails that give a negative result. In the field of cancer research, only 6 of 53 landmark studies could be proven valid, meaning over ninety percent were flawed while passed off to the public as fact.[14]

While medical cancer treatments of chemotherapy, radiation, and surgery do little to prolong life, choosing to do nothing prolongs the lives of cancer patients by four times versus choosing treatment.[15] When information is withheld in a culture of secrecy, people get hurt. Tragically, forty-two percent of Americans are affected by medical mistakes, where no one is accountable.[16]

Most people are simply unaware that they carry their own healing medicine within—their immune system—to heal and reverse disease.

> *There is no need to 'stimulate' the immune system, as many [pharmaceutical] immune therapies today attempt to do; the immune system is designed and optimized to repair any dysfunction on its own … Once the proper support is supplied to the immune system, it awakens and acts with a speed and power that can only be termed awesome to behold.*
> *— Dr. Nicholas Gonzalez, Vitality Magazine[17]*

Many people who successfully reverse cancer do so naturally, by working with their cells, not against them. Evidence shows that cancer cells thrive because they have unlocked an ancestral toolkit of pre-existing, supportive adaptations to reinvent themselves. This is not the Darwinian theory of evolution we all learned about in school.[18] We can learn from the wisdom of our own cells.

Cancer cells are your cells adapting to survive a hostile bodily environment. The sad truth is that when we spend trillions of dollars to wage chemical and nuclear war to destroy "rogue" cancer cells, we fail to see a complex and natural process of cell cooperation. "Immortal" cancer cells have selected traits they carry with them that resist death. Cells are not genetically programmed to die, as in apoptosis, rather they are programmed to survive ongoing abuse of an inhospitable milieu that changes the genes into the cancer personality type.

Where did we go wrong in our thinking?

During Francis Galton's time, ideas were shifting, as ideas tend to do. In the 1860s, Louis Pasteur developed his Germ Theory of Disease, which created a fear of an invisible, external agent—the germ. Suddenly, people felt powerless over their own bodies. Soon after that, orthodox medicine edged out natural medicine under the controlling interests of the Rockefeller Institute of Medical Research funded by the Federal Reserve Bank (FED), established in 1913.

A few individuals in high places began a public relations campaign to manipulate the social habits and opinions of the people as a way to engineer consent. The term "public health" created the "herd" to replace individual health, while the "deadly virus" displaced the all-powerful immune system. The dualistic "us vs. them" mentality held. The public mindset served to drive the illness deeper into the body to create a more serious condition, while driving the patient to become a lifelong customer of the medical industrial complex.

As if wearing blindfolds, together we have allowed humanity to be led and misled through the manipulation of science and of our psyches. While science has been used for good, it has also been used to program and deceive. As a result, science should always be questioned. However, under fear-based campaigns we lose our curiosity. Out of fear we are disempowered. We are allergic to taking responsibility for our lives and afraid to trust ourselves. Instead we ask for permission and, in the process, we become slaves of a system to which we consent.

If we are to take back our health, we must take back our minds, unplug from false theories, and withdraw consent. We can return to the wisdom of the body. Nature liberates us to align body, mind, soul, and spirit so the healing process can begin. In Nature, there is no separation, no duality, no self and other, no opposition, no conflict and no destruction. The ancient elements of Nature were regarded as the elements of life and survival before they were reduced to their atomic properties. Each has its own personality and essence.

Of Nature's elements, the iodine archetype represents the holistic view missing in the science of today. Iodine's personality is one of compassion, laughter, humanitarianism, and liberation for victims who suffer. From this larger view, we not only see how an iodine imbalance creates victimhood, but also how we can naturally reverse this condition by replenishing lost iodine reserves.

On the path from victimhood to freedom it is pivotal for each of us to accept responsibility for our bodies. Health is not found in any orthodoxy or system. We free ourselves to heal by trusting intuition to find our own answers. Health, like happiness, is an inside job and a birthright. No one else is authorized to hold the keys to our bodies unless consent is given. By our divine nature, we create our own health and heal our own disease.

The world shows up according to how we view it.
— *Eliot Cowan, Plant Spirit Medicine*

In his book *Plant Spirit Medicine*, shaman Eliot Cowan states that whether we choose a dualistic view or whether we choose a nondualistic view—where we are a part of everything—we prove our view correct when we act on it. Each view has its potential and its limitations based on the psyche, or ego, of each individual. However, we must also remember we have a soul and a spirit. Dualism ignores the spirit and thus, alienates us from our very selves.

Under holism, we are in relationship with spirit to see disease as the opportunity to heal on higher and higher levels. The spirit of Nature teaches, "balance in everything" as it evolves to higher dimensions.

Our "woe is me" state of dependency is a wake-up call. There is no need to "live with thyroid disease" when you can break free to heal yourself. The moment you stop attacking yourself is the moment antibodies (anti-self) cease to exist.

When you focus attention to healing vs. disease you begin to replenish your reserves. If you don't invest in yourself, who will? If you don't love and respect yourself, why should anyone else? As soon as you decide to love yourself, you claim your inheritance as a healer. If I was able to reverse thyroid disease naturally, so can you.

Chapter One

Voice

There is a voice inside of you
That whispers all day long,
"I feel this is right for me,
I know that this is wrong."
No teacher, preacher, parent, friend
Or wise man can decide
What's right for you—just listen to
The voice that speaks inside.

— *Shel Silverstein*

How many times do you fail to speak up when offered the opportunity? Do you question the authenticity of your voice? Is it easier to let others speak for you? Do you self-censor in favor of keeping the peace? What if I suggested that if you are able to free your voice and speak your truth, you realign in a way that allows you to heal yourself, and heal your thyroid?

I'm speaking from experience. As someone who rarely spoke up, who dreaded public speaking throughout my educational career, I grew up choosing to express myself through classical ballet and creative writing. By the time I started a family and chose to stay home to raise my kids, I thought I had successfully circumnavigated the matter, only to discover I'd shut down my thyroid.

Today, the thyroid disease epidemic affects four out of ten people, and more than 200 million worldwide.[19] Hypothyroidism goes undiagnosed in at least fifty percent of cases.[20] The fact is, if you are a woman between the ages of 20 and 40, you can almost hear the word *hypothyroidism* ringing in your ear.

While medical research has focused solely on the physical body, disease rates continue to climb. Medicine fails to go beneath the surface to uncover all of our qualities—body, mind, soul, and spirit—to understand the hidden causes of imbalance. In my own search for profound healing, I traveled to the depths and ultimately found my voice.

People talk about 'finding your voice,' but it's bigger than that because you're participating in it. It's not just looking and hoping and waiting for voice to arrive. What you're saying and how you're saying it merge. And one feeds into the other. Qualities of the voice emerge that are bigger than what you were used to. It's more. More power is being expressed in different ways. It's healing. It's art. It's so many things all wrapped up into one. Voice.

— Jon Rappoport, personal interview

Your voice is your music deep within, that is being called out. Voice reverberates through water, which makes up more than three-quarters of your body. Voice communicates through sound, which can also mean a bay or a channel. Sound turns energy into form, using certain frequency patterns that attract energy to flow in predictable ways. These patterns are sacred geometries that are the building blocks of matter, as revealed in the science of cymatics, which make sound visible. You feel your voice in your gut and in your bones, and through every cell of your being. When voice speaks through the heart, its language is love, and its message is truth.

Truth is individual, based on perception. There is always more than one truth. As perception changes and consciousness expands, support for old paradigms falls apart and we are able to see and act on new truths. To find truth is to resonate with a specific frequency, not unlike tuning into a radio station. Therefore, debating truth is conflict because truth is relative, at the level of ego. The deepest truth is love and love does not require any defense.

What if we had learned, as children, that truth lives in the domain of the heart as an expression of the divine? The ultimate truth, then, is to trust what you know deep inside, even if others attempt to convince you otherwise. The hardest thing to do when others call you crazy is to trust your inner truth, but that is what you came here to do. The only real truth is the truth that is self-realized, deep within the core of your being. Your truth is your inner voice, the language of your soul. Trust it.

If we are each individual expressions of divinity, then we can appreciate who we are on a higher level. *Appreciate* means to increase in value. We are the value. What each of us brings into motion with our choices transforms all of us. What if we had learned to simply stand in our individual truths and give voice to it?

Truth communicates as your Inner Child, your spirit. Your spirit is the spark that separates you from the rest of the crowd. Spirit expresses as passion and compassion, purpose and perseverance, patience and tolerance. Feelings are the language of spirit. So even when you hold back your voice, spirit is always nudging and guiding you. No matter how deeply your voice is buried, if it is allowed a clear path of expression, it can be used to heal.

For the writer, voice finds expression through words, for the dancer, through movement, for the painter, through color, and for the musician, through song. As an artist, your voice is your instrument, playing in harmony with nature. Allow it air and space to breathe. Let it take shape. Practice your instrument and do not abandon it. Speak your truth and tell it like it is. When you finally choose to hear your own voice, you might just wake up to yourself.

Hermann Hesse, German poet and novelist whose works portrayed an individual's spiritual search, wrote, "There is no reality except the one contained within us. That is why so many people live such an unreal life. They take the images outside them for reality and never allow the world within to assert itself."[21]

Hesse's ideas strike a chord with a basic truth. When we suppress who we are physically, mentally, emotionally, and spiritually—when we fail to speak our truth—we fall into dis-ease. Just as suppressing physical symptoms with drugs drives a toxin deeper into the body to do greater damage overtime, so, too, does suppressing the gift of your voice.

Any disease, like our reality, stems from our own making. *Life is what we make of it.* To make our music, we must not only attune to our voice but also attune to our unique truth. By honing the voice, we each offer our unique gift to the world.

Whether we expand into health or contract into disease, we manifest the physical body from the coherence or dissonance of our music. If the voice inside says we are not good enough, we believe it, create it, and live it. It becomes a pattern that plays out in all areas of life, work, and play.

> *Watch your thoughts, for they become words. Watch your words, for they become actions. Watch your actions, for they become habits. Watch your habits, for they become character. Watch your character, for it becomes your destiny.*
> — *Author Unknown*

If you believe no one finds you beautiful, because you compare yourself to others, you project that view onto the world, and you see it reflected it back to you in how others behave toward you. Breaking old patterns means your perception must shift, and that requires imagination. Nobel Physicist Max Planck said, "When you change the way you look at things, the things you look at change."

> *"The imagination works on the threshold that runs between light and dark, visible and invisible, quest and question, possibility and fact. The imagination is the great friend of possibility. Where the imagination is awake and alive, fact never hardens or closes but remains open, inviting you to new thresholds of possibility and creativity."*
> — *Anam Cara, A book of Celtic Wisdom*

Imagination asks, "What if?" It is a combination of desires, intentions, and fears. It is thinking, dreaming, and picturing. It is you interpreting reality. Imagination can trick you or liberate you. Your unique view is based in imagination, which generates beliefs, thoughts, intentions, words, and emotions. Emotions are the sum total of your wealth as a healer. Emotions are the trigger and they are managed by your own endocrine system.

Endocrine System
⬇

Beliefs ➡ Thoughts ➡ Emotions ➡ Words ➡ Actions ➡ Reality

E-motion is energy in motion

E-MOTION
Emotions are energy in motion, or e-motion. They generate chemical releases that produce physical effects, directed by your

5

endocrine system. When undigested emotions, like undigested food, become stuck in the body, they block energy flow, which can lead to a low-functioning thyroid and result in weight gain. In other words, symptoms that manifest are a perfect expression of emotions you suppress.

Like words, thoughts and emotions resonate as sound frequencies in your cells. Your cell receptors contain mini antennae able to read energy fields to alter a protein's charge on the cell membrane. A shift in charge causes the receptor to change shape in order to allow in or repel other charged molecules. When you hold a feeling, you hold a vibratory pattern that is stored in your physical organs that literally changes your biology. This is the science of epigenetics—the science of change. It explains how interactions with our environment such as diet, sleep patterns, toxic exposures, and emotions turn genes on and off.[22]

All that emotional momentum has to go somewhere. Anger, frustration, and bitterness migrate to the liver and gallbladder. Fear and anxiety go to the bladder and kidneys. Grief goes to the lungs. Loss of power or responsibility finds the pancreas. Excess in any form goes to the heart. Lack of joy goes to the thyroid.

People with thyroid problems tend to be shy, timid, and insecure. They avoid conflict at all costs. They often distract themselves with obligations. They feel choked or blocked when trying to express themselves. They worry what others will think. They are hesitant to share themselves, their beliefs, their life choices, and often feel they have to hide who they really are. They bury their emotions. They feel they don't have a voice. They are martyrs.

In her book, *You Can Heal Your Life*, Louise Hay suggests people with thyroid conditions suffer from feelings of humiliation. Goiter, an enlarged thyroid, reflects feelings of victimization and powerlessness that can eventually lead to cancer. Hypothyroidism mirrors hopelessness and suffocation. Hyperthyroidism stems from rage at being left out. In each case, the cure is in understanding that these are negative thought patterns that no longer serve your mission or highest potential.

Resistance pinches off the flow of energy where fear is the driving force. Fear hides behind emotions we would rather ignore—inadequacy, worthlessness, and emptiness. Fear is a sign of disconnection from Self. However, all negative emotions have their place and purpose. They point us to the areas inside that need love, the areas that have been fragmented or shut down from past experiences in order to cope. If we can move forward without fear then there is no resistance and no need for discomfort or disease.

Attitude is the difference between an ordeal and an adventure.
— *Author Unknown*

In the adventure called life, most of us will be challenged with an ordeal. A painful event will cause us to question our purpose. Passion fades. We lose energy. We come out of balance. We contract. We can't breathe. Whether the event was the death of a loved one or the death of something inside of us, we are left numb with feelings of despair, unworthiness, abandonment, or loss. Though the ordeal may be different for each of us, none of us escapes it.

Our emotional wounds are stories. They contain lessons and show us the solutions if we are open to reading them. Our shadows, like our light, are parts that want to be seen, validated, and integrated. Where light is information, darkness is ignorance. To bring light to the darkness is not easy if fear overrides. But you can start by asking yourself what you would have to believe about yourself in order to feel the way you do. Listen for the answer. Use your imagination.

The Inka shamans believe there are no "bad" energies, only "light" that supports life and "heavy" energies that cannot be digested. "Everything living is light bound into matter," says shaman Alberto Villoldo in his book, *Shaman, Healer, Sage.* The heavy, toxic energies that congest a chakra fuel emotional imprints and must be combusted and metabolized. Like a log in a fire, once the light is released, the imprints of disease are cleared. The ashes are taken back into the earth to be transformed and the light is reabsorbed into the body.

LETTING GO

In healing, it is critical to let go of the things you have been grasping onto so tightly, whether they are fears, beliefs, situations, or people. Do not compromise yourself in order to elevate others. You may need to walk away from insecure people to rise to your highest potential. Letting go means being honest with yourself so you can live in integrity and authenticity. It means listening to your truth in favor of other's opinions. It means trusting your process.

> *By letting go, it all gets done. The world is won by those who let it go. But when you try and try, the world is beyond winning.*
> — *Lao-Tzu*

In the film *The Wizard of Oz*, Dorothy faces a crisis that sets her on a spiritual journey. She escapes over the rainbow and spirals from her outer world of Kansas to fall into her inner world of Oz, connected to the same cast of characters acting as her alter egos. In Oz she longs for her true home but is told by the great Wizard of Oz that she must go on a scavenger hunt—do his dirty work—before she is able to return.

Along her path, Dorothy meets three compatriots, each reflecting an aspect of her own perceived emptiness: the Scarecrow who lacks a brain (thinking), the Tin Woodman who lacks a heart (feeling), and the Cowardly Lion who lacks courage (will). By journey's end, Dorothy discovers that the Wizard was merely an illusion—her creation—and that she always held the power to return home. Dorothy let go to live in her integrity. She claimed responsibility for herself.

The Wizard of Oz shows that "wherever you go, there you are." Crisis follows us until we are able to make a new choice, and act on it. Dorothy had courage to take her first steps on that yellow brick road without a map. But, in the end, she also had the heart and the free will necessary to release resistance to be able to come back home to her True Self. The challenge that each of us face is to let go and be swept away into the abyss of imagination where a new reality is possible. It is only when we travel to the depths, that we discover what we need to push off bottom to propel ourselves to the surface for freedom. Dorothy let go and trusted intuition.

Intuition is about coming into your own. It's the chill running up your spine, your gut feeling, your sixth sense, your inner navigator. It warns, "This doesn't add up" and advises, "Trust your feelings."

When you tap into intuition, you tap into primal instinct. The stronger your intuition, the stronger your voice. The more you trust, the more often the right answers will come. To trust that you have your own answers is to love yourself unconditionally. This is not selfish. This is self-love.

Trusting intuition involves trusting your soul as your co-pilot in making decisions. Intuition says, "see disease as an opportunity" to take inventory of your life's path. Within every problem there is a solution, a key, a medicine, a gift, a teaching, a learning, an opening. In a state of contraction there is always the opportunity for expansion.

On the other side of fear is opportunity.
— Lewis Howes, author

TRUST YOUR PROCESS

All challenges, whether breakdowns or break-ups, deaths or diagnoses, are divinely designed for the purpose of individual growth, which in turn affects the evolution of all humanity. To breakthrough the conflict of dualism, is to find the peace of nondualism.

Accept the challenge. Embrace it. See it as a gift. And let it be a source of strength. You may as well accept what is happening since all your choices brought you to this point. *Resistance is futile.* Be open to spirit and ready to receive. Be available. Show up and others will show up for you. The people you attract in your life are your teachers and mentors. They are gifts to show you the parts that need attention and healing. Though they may disagree with you, allow no one to pull you off your path no matter how adamant they are. They are just doing their job, even if they are unaware of it. They are doing an important service. They are not to blame for the dramas and challenges that arise as part of your own vibration. When you only see a deficiency, that is called self-denial, which leads to victimization of yourself or someone else. When you can separate other people's opinions from the wisdom received from mentors, and balance that wisdom with your own intuition, then you are no longer victim to someone else's ideals. The change you make can take your life to the next level.

Thyroid disease is a call from spirit through the language of your body to wake up to your own voice. Mark Twain once said, "All of us contain music and truth but most of us can't get it out." Are you ready to journey to free your voice, tell your truth, and sing your song?

Chapter Two

Backstory

I count myself as one who has emerged from a detour into the abyss. At age 44, I was diagnosed with profound hypothyroidism. I felt lost. With my family all around me, I felt alone. As someone who'd trained in the environmental health field and proactively chose a healthy lifestyle to prevent disease, I felt my disease condition had manifested out of thin air. Nothing made sense in the logical world.

Profound hypothyroidism is the Cadillac of thyroid disease. It is the most severe and acute form of hypothyroidism, when the thyroid completely shuts down and stops making thyroid hormone. As the master gland of metabolism for every cell in the body, my thyroid had put up its "Out to Lunch" sign. When that happens, the heart begins to starve.

At that point I was faced with a choice. Should I do what my doctor urged and agree to immediately take a synthetic drug, levothyroxine, known as Synthroid, for the rest of my life, and before I keeled over? Or should I listen to my gut, and do it my way? How would I proceed?

Up to this point I let others do the talking. My study of

biology and environmental health science led me to serve as an environmental scientist for the U.S. Environmental Protection Agency writing air pollution regulations. As a government employee, I followed direction and held my tongue as I observed conflicts of interest and political favors play out around me.

After three years of failing to meet my personal objectives working for an agency that generated more roadblocks than pathways to protecting human health and the environment, I traded in my badge for a stroller, started a family, and stayed home to raise my three children. Instead of writing regulations, I joined a writing group and wrote children's fiction and poetry. In place of protecting "public health," I focused on my children's health and breathed a sigh of relief because I believed I'd successfully navigated my fear of speaking. I thought I was home free.

And then all hell broke loose. With my health in decline and a diagnosis of profound hypothyroidism in hand, I realized that in my effort to suppress my voice, I'd completely shut down my thyroid.

Ironically, the thyroid had been a subject of interest for me long before my diagnosis. I had been researching the thyroid to help a friend naturally reverse her own diagnosis of hyperthyroidism. Natural healing has been a passion since childhood as I watched my father deliberately use herbal therapies to avoid his doctor's prescriptions. He lived to the age of ninety-four in his own home, gardening vegetables and eating my mother's home cooking. What he knew about botanicals came from growing up in India raised by his mother, the village healer, who found medicinal plants right outside her front door. While my siblings, my husband, father-in-law, and one grandfather identified as allopathic medical doctors, I chose the path of my Indian roots.

Four years prior to my diagnosis, in an attempt to prevent what I saw as an epidemic of thyroid disease showing up in my friends as they turned forty, I began prophylactically supplementing with Lugol's iodine. While I had silently declared that thyroid disease would not find me, here I sat, reluctantly, branded with the most severe form.

Shaman and author Robert Moss writes, "Such obstruction isn't random, and it's about more than toughening us up. Dead ends and adversity, repeated often enough, can make us aware that we've been following the wrong charts. Knowing that we have been misdirected gives us the chance to find our true direction."[23] His words rang true. My diagnosis was a clarion call showing me that I had bypassed the direction of my calling. It asked me to reevaluate my navigational charts, to look deeper, and place myself as the beacon to turn toward.

So, with a strong signal from my gut, and against my doctor's wishes, I refused his prescription and told him that I would reverse my condition 'au natural.' No medical interventions for me, except my request for a temporary natural thyroid hormone, Armour Thyroid, to stabilize my body and allow me to "hover" while I did my own research. I would next request additional antibody testing to confirm autoimmunity so I could tweak my diet if necessary.

RESEARCH & CHARTING THE COURSE FORWARD

Autoimmune thyroiditis, also known as Hashimoto's, had eventually been confirmed, but not from my medical doctor who refused my request for antibody testing. In his words, "Why would I test for autoimmunity when it won't change the way I treat you?" His comment spoke to his inability to work outside a system of disease-based codes, pre-approved tests, and escalating costs. What my doctor could offer was limited by what the insurance company allowed him to offer. When it comes to treatment, doctors are hamstrung.

Years before I was diagnosed, I was employed at the Mayo Clinic as a cytogenetics lab technologist. I was told to get the Hepatitis B vaccine series over a six month period to "protect myself" against accidental viral infection from possible needle sticks. Later, in graduate school, I

13

agreed to a measles vaccine booster. Only months later did I connect these series of shots to a case of pneumonia and frequent bouts of bronchitis from the suppression of my immune system.

As a mother who saw similar pathologies play out in my children after receiving vaccines, I sat before my doctor, with hindsight, supported by my file of medical references. I made a request for antibody testing to rule out autoimmune disease. The doctor stared at his computer. "I don't have the time to look at your research and I won't order more tests," he said. He would not discuss nutritional approaches. He said no to antibody testing. And he believed that iodine supplementation I had utilized caused thyroid disease in all cases.[24] Our universes collided. My intuition told me that this doctor suffered from a deficiency of knowledge and a closed mind.

What I came to realize, in time, was that my doctor's response was a blessing in disguise. He motivated me to trust my gut, exit the insurance-backed medical system, and seek out someone who didn't see me as part of the herd, someone who believed, like I did, that full thyroid function could return if the body was provided with the right tools.

> *The most dangerous thing you can have is really good medical insurance.*
> — *Robert Scott Bell, The Robert Scott Bell Show*

My new functional medicine doctor performed the tests I requested, no questions asked, and no insurance accepted. The functional medical tests expanded the range of imbalance to a more realistic scope. Tests results indicated:

- Greater than fifty percent deficiency in iodine, even though I had been supplementing with Lugol's iodine solution for four years.

- High levels of bromide, a halogen, which blocks iodine from entering the cells.
- High levels of barium, tungsten, and strontium from air pollution.[25]
- High levels of thyroid antibodies TPO and Tg, confirming autoimmunity.

I phoned iodine researcher Dr. Flechas to consult with him on the question of removing my dental mercury amalgams. His information suggested that my daily iodine dose of 10 drops of Lugol's iodine was adequate in pulling the mercury out of the body and into the urine, and recommended not to force the issue, "if it isn't broken don't fix it." For the other metals, he recommended that I retake the metals test later to verify the metals are at undetectable levels. Eventually, I chose to remove my dental amalgams with a biological dentist over several visits to reduce my body burden.

METAL HAVOC

Viruses alone do not cause autoimmunity. Viruses, parasites, yeast overgrowth, and other pathogenic microbes are a measure of health on a disease continuum. They are present due to metal toxicity from environmental exposures, such as mercury from dental fillings, copper from DDT in soil, and aluminum from vaccines. Many metals are inhaled from atmospheric fallout of the government cloud-seeding programs begun in the 1950s. Programs, such as The Manhattan Project, aerosolized nanoparticles of barium, strontium, and other metals that continue worldwide under geo-engineering programs.[26] According to the 2018 CDC vaccine schedule, babies in the first 15 months of life received twenty-two doses of eleven vaccines, with each dose containing an aluminum adjuvant. During the first 18 months of life, babies are injected with 4,925 µg of aluminum.[31] Metals cause inflammation in the gut, which travel through the blood-brain barrier to cause inflammation in the brain. They remain in the body when the eliminatory organs—liver, kidneys, colon, lungs, lymphatic fluid—fail to function optimally due to congestion. For instance, mercury in vaccines binds to glutathione to dismantle the body's ability to remove metals. Mercury also blocks selenium-dependent enzymes needed for thyroid hormone conversion.

Professor Christopher Exley of Keele University in England found dangerously high levels of aluminum in the brains of children diagnosed with autism, who died from encephalitis. Encephalitis is listed as an adverse reaction in vaccine package inserts.[27] The only other brains observed containing similar levels of aluminum died from Alzheimer's disease[28]—two ends of a toxic metal spectrum disorder.

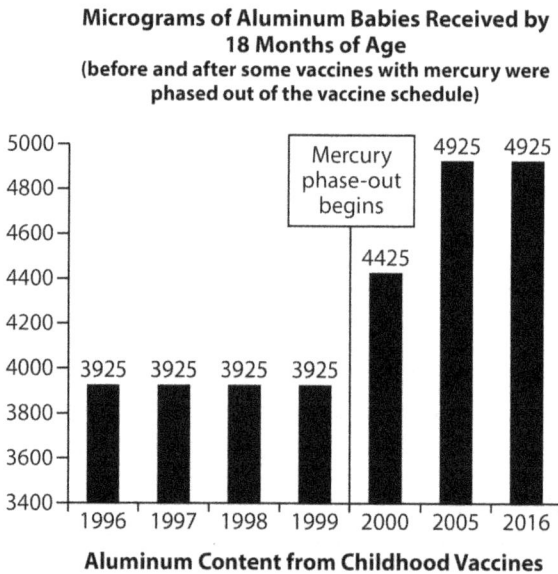

Microgrms of Aluminum Babies Received by 18 Months of Age
(before and after some vaccines with mercury were phased out of the vaccine schedule)

Aluminum Content from Childhood Vaccines

Image reproduced with permission from **Aluminum in Childhood Vaccines is Unsafe** by Neil Z. Miller, *Journal of American Physicians and Surgeons* Volume 21 Number 4 Winter 2016. Copyright ©NZM.

Figure No. 1

Aluminum adjuvants in vaccines can induce the neurological symptoms of thyroid disease and all autoimmune diseases,[29] including the chronic co-infections of Autism Spectrum Disorder and Alzheimer's disease.[30] Why do we allow it? How do we help the body remove aluminum?

Professor Chris Exley writes:

> I have been studying and researching the biology of silicon for more than 30 years and there is only one way that silicon can influence aluminium toxicity in the body and that is through its actions as silicic acid, not silica. Silica taken orally will release very small amounts of silicic acid but in the main it will move through the gut unchanged to be excreted in the faeces. Silica is a very 'sticky' substance, which means that many things in the gut may adsorb to its surfaces and thus it may help to remove gut contents via the faeces.
>
> Silicon in silicon-rich mineral waters, is in the form of silicic acid which essentially follows water throughout the body being excreted eventually in the urine and also in sweat. If you drink a silicon-rich mineral water on a regular basis, for example 1L/day, then your body fluids will equilibrate to a higher level of silicic acid then would normally be the case and provide a constant protection against the possible toxicity of aluminium.
>
> — Dr. Christopher Exley, Professor[31]

Metals are the favorite food of parasites. Today, parasites are epidemic in humans. But, they are there as beneficial helpers to remove the body's toxic metal body burden. Parasites, however, also produce neurotoxins that lead to symptoms that overlap with known symptoms of hypothyroidism. Parasites inflame the lining of the intestine by their very presence. They also create toxic byproducts from their waste and dead bodies.

Metals and toxic byproducts of pathogens cause the body's

terrain to become acidic, causing beneficial microbes to shift to pathogenic microbes. An acid gut means less acid in the stomach. Therefore, poor digestion. Poor digestion leads to poor absorption of minerals such as iron, copper, zinc, and vitamins such as A, D, and E through the gut wall. Poor absorption leads to low mineral uptake, which can indicate a methylation problem.

A methylation defect prevents the absorption of trace minerals, blocks metabolic pathways and the conversion of micronutrients, and prevents toxins from being carried out of the body. Because poor absorption leads to malnutrition, it is important not only to reintroduce missing nutrients but also to detoxify metals.

IODINE AND MINERALS

What medical doctors don't know can hurt you. Doctors fail to understand the cause of hypothyroid symptoms because they do not understand that the body works at the level of cellular energy. They fail to see that poor circulation, poor memory, and poor digestion are symptoms of poor metabolism, which is the lack of heat and energy due to a lack of iodine at the cell.

Iodine restores heat and increases the assimilation of salts for metabolism. In fact, iodine works with many minerals to keep operations running smoothly, such as phosphorous to oxidize toxic materials that affect the brain. Iodine works with boron in the parathyroid glands to prevent cataracts and bone spurs. Boron also removes fluoride so iodine can bind to its receptor sites. Iodine and selenium convert thyroid hormones. Combined with oxygen, iodine triggers cell apoptosis to allow the body to cleanse itself naturally.[32] All minerals work together for the whole. When one mineral goes missing, the body compensates by taking from other areas until operations break down and come to a stop.

Holistic doctors understand that each person has a unique biochemical balance when it comes to trace minerals and not all people use iodine from the same foods in the same way.

Whether the thyroid is labeled *hypo* or *hyper*, it lacks minerals. Without studying nutrition, medical doctors claim that iodine supplementation causes an overproduction of thyroid hormone to cause hyperthyroidism. This is a myth based on my own experience of hypothyroidism while supplementing daily for four years with 8 drops of Lugol's Solution (5% iodine).

For centuries, holistic doctors have utilized iodine supplementation to stop the thyroid from burning itself out. When absorbed, iodine creates iodolipids, which throw water on the flames. After all, iodine is a main component in the formation of thyroid hormone. Iodine is the very elixir necessary to satisfy the thyroid's thirst. Since iodine is water soluble, it enters the lymph fluids and travels to every cell in the body. My confidence in utilizing iodine came directly from books by board-certified family physician Dr. David Brownstein who uses iodine in his Michigan practice to successfully reduce or eliminate the need for thyroid hormones for his patients.

BACK TO THE BACKSTORY

Once autoimmune thyroiditis had been confirmed I began making a few changes. First, I switched to a wheat-free, gluten-free diet. Unless sprouted from seeds, wheat creates acidity due to glyphosate, an herbicide sprayed on wheat as a desiccant. Glyphosate locks up nutrients that prevent iodine from being carried into cells. It locks up chromium needed to activate insulin, and cobalt needed to make vitamin B-12. It was easy enough to remove wheat from my food plan and replace it with ancient grains, including millet, and flax.

Next, I switched from tap water to spring water to avoid chlorine and fluoride, toxic halogens that prevent iodine uptake by the thyroid. The halogens fluorine, chlorine, and bromine have a greater affinity for thyroid cell receptor sites than iodine because they are more electronegative.

Then I chose my health-support team: a functional medicine doctor, an herbal doctor, an energy healer, my yoga instructor, and my farmer. Using food as my medicine, I listened to 'the doctor within' by eating nutrient-rich, whole, non-GMO, organic, foods. My farmer provided me with organic vegetables, grass-fed meat, bones for broth, cod liver oil for fat-soluble vitamins, grass-fed raw milk, and colostrum. I had the tools to begin to heal a damaged gut.

To support digestion, detoxify the liver, and nourish the blood, I alternated between several herbs, dosed as capsules and extracts, including dandelion root, burdock root, yellow dock root, and Oregon grape root. I used black walnut hulls and kelp to cleanse yeast and support the liver and kidneys. I added methylated B-vitamins for the nervous system and blood, and liquid chlorophyll to help draw out metals. I added selenium tablets made from whole foods to avoid synthetic isolates, to detox metals such as mercury, and for selenium's potent anti-oxidant properties. I added blackstrap molasses to replace lost minerals (more on Food as Medicine in chapter ten).

After several months of eliminating wheat and tap water, while replenishing lost nutrients, my antibodies diminished and I began to feel better. With the help of the natural thyroid hormone, my thyroid hormone levels stabilized. The brain fog rolled away and my body stopped retaining water. With kelp and co-nutrients, I pushed out bromine so iodine could lock-and-load to my cell receptors. As a result, I experienced "bromide acne." This common effect of bromide detoxing through the skin told me that my liver and lymph needed further support. Since then I have experienced the benefits of the coffee enema as the easiest, cheapest, and fastest way to cleanse the liver when used in conjunction with the added nutrients of green juicing. When you extract the juice of green vegetables such as celery, cucumber, carrots, beet, and cilantro, you introduce high levels of phytonutrients, micronutrients, and enzymes in an efficient way. Juicing allows you bypass a weakened digestive system to deliver nutrients directly to cells, thereby increasing energy and allowing your body's immune system to heal.

Comfortable with my progress, I returned to the medical system under the care of a new family practice doctor who didn't question my research and actually agreed with my assessment. He asked me to put my research away because he didn't need to be convinced and would help me in any way he could. He also agreed to my only two requests: to monitor my progress through blood work as proof of my eventual disease reversal, and to accept a hug after I achieved success. Unlike my last doctor, he engendered confidence. He had my back. He believed that I would reverse my imbalance because he believed in me.

In setting my intention to participate in my own healing, I saw my world sending me confirmation through people coming into my life. I opened a window to allow someone who reflected my view of healing to walk through the door. In edging out what I would not tolerate, I manifested an amazing support team of caregivers. Next, I would need to take inventory of my life to understand why this condition manifested and why now?

CHAPTER THREE

WHAT IS AUTOIMMUNE DISEASE, REALLY?

Physicians describe thyroid autoimmunity as the body waging war against itself in a battle to the death. The literature describes T-cells as "tricked" into classifying cells as invaders. B-cells then produce antibodies to counter-attack those cells. Antibodies, or 'aggressor cells,' then launch an attack against a thyroid enzyme protein called *thyroid peroxidase* to destroy thyroid cells. Is the body really on a mission of aggression and self-sabotage through the creation of autoantibodies? Hardly.

Autoimmune thyroiditis is inflammation of the thyroid. Inflammation is due to toxemia, a condition in which a toxin —whether from junk food, microbes, products of metabolism, chemicals, metals, or a compacted colon—moves through the blood and deeper into the body. The snowball effect of toxemia changes the pH of the body's terrain and depletes minerals, which results in a shift in our microbes from beneficial to pathogenic. The body is responding exactly as designed, as a barometer of what is happening in the terrain. The Terrain Theory of Disease says the germ is not the cause of disease. The germ is a product of a shifting terrain.

In truth, the body's immune system does not go after the tissue or organ itself; rather, it responds to the microbial changes within.[33] The reason immune T-cells are called into action is not because they are tricked but because they are responding to duty, hot on the trail of a virus or bacterium. As the 2004 *Journal Nature Reviews Cancer* reports, the Epstein-Barr Virus (EBV) —a herpes virus— was found to be "widespread in all human populations and to persist in the vast majority of individuals as a lifelong asymptomatic infection of the B-lymphocyte pool."[34]

Anthony William, author of *Medical Medium*, believes the body may be going after EBV. He is partially right. Out of the roughly 320 million people in the U.S., over 225 million Americans have some form of EBV. Medical doctors recognize only one version of EBV, though there are over 60 known varieties. Medical tests are not sensitive enough to identify specific viruses, though a decline in thyroid hormone has been reported in the scientific literature as a result of bacterial infection.[35] Most doctors have no idea why the virus is there in the first place to understand the true cause of disease.

> *Western mythology tells us that we live in a predatory universe where we are constantly being stalked by "bad" microbes and hungry jaguars. Medicine people, on the other hand believe that we live in a benign universe. The world becomes predatory only when we are out of balance.*
> —*Alberto Villoldo, Shaman, Healer, Sage*

We are in relationship with our microbes as an integrated ecosystem. When our immune system is balanced, we all thrive. When it fails, we fail. Because we are interdependent, we must work together with our microbes for our mutual survival. The best way to appreciate our microbes is to understand them on their level by unveiling the lost Law of the Terrain.

LAW OF THE TERRAIN

Under the Law of the Terrain, our cells, microbes, and our viruses work together. They depend on minerals from our food and water just as we depend on them. Humans embody both a microbiome and a virome, showing that our microbes are critical companions in the delicate balance in every layer of our innate immune system, so it makes sense to get to know them on an intimate level.

Up to 40,000 different bacterial species, or one trillion beneficial bacteria, live in the one-celled, mucosal epithelial lining of the digestive tract, which stretches from mouth to anus. The "gut" is the microbiome, considered the center of the immune system, where our microbes outnumber our own cells 10 to 1. In fact, every organ system has its own microbiome with its own unique species. Thus, the microbes on the skin are different from those in the stomach. Our microbes determine how we feel, how we age, how large or thin we are, and whether we are susceptible to depression, bipolar disorder, anxiety, or not. When our microbes are not happy, we feel it. When they are ill, so are we. The sheer diversity of microbes illustrates the extent to which these bugs work to ensure their own survival. We are also four percent virus. Bugs R Us. In the right ratio, our microbes are the gatekeepers to true health for body and mind.

Because our bugs connect the gut-brain axis, imbalances in gut bacteria can lead to depression and obsessive-compulsive disorder.[36] Damage to our mucosal lining from antibiotics, vaccines, drugs, radiation, toxins, and/or stress that causes digestive distress also stops neural growth in the hippocampus, the area associated with memory.[37] Our bugs go beyond the body. They connect us to Earth and sky. The same bacteria that live in our skin, in our blood, and in our cells also inhabit the soil. They are found in a glacial core sample and also in the upper troposphere, ten kilometers above the Earth's surface.[38] Our inherent connection to our environment was revealed in the late 1960s by biologist Lynn Margulis who showed that our own mitochondrial cells are both primitive bacteria and chloroplasts living in synergy to supply energy and produce food from sunlight.

In public school, we do not learn that we are a microbiome and a virome living symbiotically with Earth; that we are both caretakers of our bodies and keepers of Earth. We are not taught that microbes working in the soil perform the same jobs in our bodies; that they help process our food, provide for our defense, and remove the garbage. We learn the hard way that what we do to the Earth, we do to ourselves.

Two centuries ago, in 1870, Claude Bernard and Antoine Bechamp, two adversaries of Louis Pasteur and his Germ Theory, revealed the Law of the Terrain. They considered germs to be the scavengers of disease, not the cause. Germs appeared when the body's natural metabolic processes were thrown off.

Looking through his microscope, Antoine Bechamp observed that when conditions of the terrain shifted—pH, nutritional status, toxicity—so did the microorganisms. To adapt, the bacterium shape-shifted to diverse stages of itself without losing its essence as it worked in harmony with its surroundings. The scene playing out was one of cooperation not victimization. Bernard devoted his life to prove the vital unity of all organisms.

Later, in 1925, Dr. Enderlein described this shape-shifting microbe as the "endobiont" which evolves to higher valence states— from normal to bacterial to fungal. As it evolves, its waste products poison human body fluids to produce a new stage of disease. When the body becomes chronically stressed due to chemical pollution and toxins, cells can no longer take up oxygen efficiently and shift, from aerobic to anaerobic metabolism, to become acidic.

Cancer grows in oxygen deprived acidic tissue. Disease cannot live in an alkaline body.
— Dr. Otto Heinrich Warburg, Nobel Prize winner

Harvey Bigelsen, M.D., author of *Holographic Blood*, wrote, "disease is a living process." Cancer reflects a fungal adaptation due to the presence of accumulated metals and radiation. Fungus or mold reflects an adaptation to an acidic terrain. Cutting out cancer does not prevent mold from growing back. If mold is in the body, it is there for a reason. As the process progresses, and all internal resources are exhausted, the mold begins to consume the organism.

Our bacteria wear many hats. They reflect the universal story of life, adaptation, death, and rebirth. When conditions of the terrain are optimal, an endobiont reverts back to its natural state. Antoine Bechamp called this process *pleiomorphism*. The endobiont doesn't die. It simply adapts. Different types of microbes are merely different manifestations of a bacterial whole always working to adapt to its environment. The problem arises when microbes enter the body unnaturally and en masse.

If a virus enters the body unnaturally, it does so through the Trojan Horse of bundled vaccines. Vaccines are considered "biologics" since they contain foreign organisms—viruses bacteria, mycoplasms, bovine protein, aborted fetal cells, as well as antibiotics, aspartame, MSG, formaldehyde, chemicals, and metals, including the adjuvant aluminum—which hyperstimulate the immune system.

A 2017 Italian study revealed the alarming presence of micro- and nano-sized particles and inorganic matter in vaccines not declared on the label. Once injected, these foreign bodies—lead, stainless steel, tungsten, cerium, iron, titanium, nickel— which are neither biodegradable, nor biocompatible induce an inflammatory reaction that leads to an autoimmune reaction.[39] Metals are the trigger.

Since these ingredients and their contaminants are injected directly into muscle and blood, they bypass the protective barriers of the skin and mucosal layers of the immune system. The immune system is balanced between two poles: 1) cellular or T cell-mediated immunity, and 2) humoral or B cell-mediated immunity, and they have a reciprocal relationship. When one is artificially stimulated, the other is suppressed.

When viruses are injected into the body, an imbalance occurs—only B cells are activated to create antibodies. Killer T cells are subsequently inhibited, and some types of virus can temporarily inactivate killer T cells. Dr. Rebecca Carley, M.D. writes, "The 'prevention' of a disease via vaccination is, in reality, an inability to expel organisms due to the suppression of the cell-mediated response. Thus, rather than preventing disease, the disease is actually prevented from ever being resolved."[40]

Natural, life-long immunity from natural infection, such as measles, whooping cough, mumps, and influenza, creates a partnership between the two poles of immunity to prevent the same disease from expressing itself in the future. The body is working holistically through an extracellular matrix that acts as an organ onto itself called the interstitium.[41] Just as our bacteria are fed by the medium in which they live, so too are our cells fed and cleansed by a network of fluid-filled spaces known as the interstitium fed by lymph fluids full of white blood cells. This shows that antibodies, by themselves, do not confer immunity,[42] just as viruses are not harmful when the conditions of the terrain are balanced.

Holism explains that when people are exposed to a virus, not everyone gets sick. Researchers at the University of Michigan (U of M) showed that when injected with infectious viral agents, a strong immune system and infectious disease could not co-exist.[43] The immune system determines whether a virus manifests or not. The U of M study suggests that there is an active immune response, both antioxidant and cell-mediated, which accounts for the resistance of sickness in certain people. Both gene expression and metabolism affect whether someone gets sick or not. [44]

THE VIRUS: TO BE OR NOT TO BE?

What if the concept of the virus as the cause of disease was a PR campaign created to hide the truth about the power of the immune system?

In 1967, the Public Health Service marketed the measles vaccine as a way to eradicate the measles virus. They promoted a mass vaccination campaign in an article titled, *Epidemiologic Basis for Eradication of Measles Virus in 1967*:

> Until very recently, the deep respect for the biological balance of the human race with the measles virus had become accepted doctrine. Eradication was not considered to be scientifically tenable. All of this has now changed. With the isolation of the measles virus and the development and extensive field testing of several potent and effective vaccines, the tools are at hand to eradicate the infection. With the general application of these tools during the coming months, eradication can be achieved in this country in the year 1967.[45]

Of course, measles eradication never happened. Large measles outbreaks continue to occur in highly vaccinated populations and along with more serious complications than with natural measles infection.[46] The suppression of the immune system by a synthetic measles virus laced with metals is one explanation why the measles vaccine causes frequent and more severe allergies and autoimmune reactions.[47]

SABOTAGE BY STEALTH VIRUSES

Medicine is moving further into genome editing. Technologies under names such as CRYSPR and IGT, 'immunoprophylaxis by gene transfer', insert genes into viruses and inject them via vaccines. These foreign genes incorporate into the recipient's DNA to produce new proteins the body has never before seen.[48] Adjuvants in vaccines also contain synthetic recombinant DNA that embed foreign DNA into mammalian cells.

The Kingdom of God is within you (Luke 17:21 KJV)

When Jesus said, "The Kingdom of God is within you," he was referring to the awareness that each of us is a divine spark of God. The kingdom is invisible, beyond the physical reality of the body. It never dies. Yet, any kingdom, visible or not, can succumb to attack and corruption if defenses are not fortified.

Stealth viruses and their payloads commit espionage and sabotage of the immune system when they breach the integrity of the skin barrier, the first layer of defense. They flow unseen through blood and lymph. As invaders fail to be targeted and eliminated, they begin to take down the system from within. Foreign "plasmids" shut genes off to prevent important immune proteins, such as GC protein, from working with our macrophages. New disorders are "discovered" that provide the fodder for the campaign of a new universal flu vaccine, always to "eradicate the deadly virus."

Ironically, the clear identification of HIV,[49] influenza virus,[50] and measles virus[51] is never found when investigators go looking for them with the latest technologies. Scientists know that a virus cannot exist as a life form outside a cell. Viruses function without sensory organs and without a means of locomotion. A virus is incapable of entering the cell membrane because a virus cannot detect it.

In a 2016 ruling, the German Federal Supreme Court disproved the existence of the measles virus using genetic evidence based on two main findings:[52]

1. They have misinterpreted ordinary constituents of cells as part of the suspected measles virus. "The phenomena presented as measles viruses are actually cellular vesicles."
2. "The criterion of the claim to prove the existence of the measles virus by 'a scientific publication' was not fulfilled by the applicant."

To this day, an actual structure that corresponds to the virus model has been found neither in a human, nor in an animal. Under the

Law of the Terrain, a virus is present because the conditions of the cell's internal terrain allow it to be there. A virus is there because it has morphed—through pleiomorphism—from a previous form in order to survive the new conditions inside the cell. In *the case of the missing virus*, the curtain is being pulled back to reveal the deception of the Germ Theory of Disease.

Germ Theory (Pasteur)	Terrain Theory (Bechamp)
Disease arises from germs outside the body.	Disease arises from microbes within cells.
Shapes and colors of microbes are constant.	Shapes and colors of microbes change to reflect the environment.
Microbes are primary causal agents.	Microbes become pathogenic as health of organism deteriorates.
Disease can strike anyone.	Disease is built upon unhealthy conditions.
To prevent disease, we need vaccines.	To prevent disease we have to create health.
Every disease is associated with a specific microbe.	Every disease is associated with a particular condition.

In our blind acceptance of The Germ Theory, we have traded infectious disease for autoimmune disease. Harmless childhood infections such as measles, once known to create a robust immune system to prevent future cancers, have been reclassified as *dangerous* and *life threatening*. Today, rates of autoimmune thyroiditis and thyroid cancer skyrocket, while diseased-based medicine is a trillion dollar business model that creates its own customers. Where once synthetic medications functioned as a stopgap measure, they are now terminal, till death do us part.

Vaccines began as homeopathy. In the late 18th century, Samuel Hahnemann developed a homeopathic remedy called a nosode from the excretions of diseased skin to cure the condition. Homeopathic nosodes are essences of the original material. As vibrational medicines, they do not contain live or weakened microbes that cause the chromosomal damage that vaccines do. They do not incorporate foreign DNA and RNA that generate genetic mutations and disorders.

Just a century ago, there were 22 homeopathic medical schools, 100 homeopathic hospitals, and over 1,000 homeopathic pharmacies. Boston University, Stanford University, and New York Medical College all taught homeopathy. This all changed in 1910 due to the Flexner Report, funded by John Rockefeller and Andrew Carnegie, and others. The Flexner Report was an attempt to align medical education under a set of norms that emphasized laboratory research and the patenting of medicine. Grants were offered only to medical-based curriculums. By removing any mention of the natural healing power of herbs and plants, or of the importance of diet to health, medical education pushed out non-allopathic schools.

The goal of homeopathy is to stimulate the immune system to help the body reverse the disease process. An historical comparison shows the true benefit of homeopathy. After World War I, an estimated 50 million people died worldwide during the Spanish Influenza. The death rate of Spanish-flu patients treated with allopathic medicine was almost 30 percent, while the death rate for those treated homeopathically was 1.05 percent. Gelsemium was the remedy most commonly used. Yet today, the FDA seeks to continue the original effort to eliminate access to homeopathy and other natural remedies.

It is time to call out science for its false narratives and shaky foundations. Our true nature is always changing with respect to our surroundings. The body is the vessel of the kingdom within, and the immune system our border security. Fortification comes from an awareness of our divinity, that we are all expressions of the same consciousness. There is no enemy germ except the one that invades our minds to delude us.

Chapter Four

Spirit Medicine

What is the deeper truth of autoimmune disease? Why did I, and so many other women, create antibodies against our own cells? Why did we choose to attack ourselves? With my chosen team of healers, I was guided to go deeper into spirit medicine.

Like Dorothy, I had stepped onto the yellow brick road without a map. So I dove into the research to gain some perspective. The studies I read indicated that all hormone therapies, thyroid hormone included, increased the risk of breast cancer over time.[53] I did not intend to worsen my situation. My intention to restore my thyroid, *sans* medication, was top priority. I elected to give the natural hormone six months to help stabilize my thyroid and heart and then discontinue. Within three short months, I had my energy back, yet a tickle in my throat persisted. How would I reach the next level of healing? What was I missing?

Meeting with the new medical doctor, I asked if he had any thoughts I hadn't considered. He said I should begin working with my gifts. On the back of his pad, he scribbled his prescription— "Hands of Light" by Barbara Ann Brennan, a book on energy healing.

This medical doctor was my first encounter with a teacher of the healing arts. *Doctor* in Latin means *teacher*. This doctor was a bridge who set the stage for the shift that was to follow. Not too long after my meeting with him, a friend introduced me to the works of several spiritual authors who wrote about a heart-based connection to spirit. As I read, I learned a new language. These writers became my daily companions.

The inner work had begun. But my greatest challenge would be letting go of expectations, especially my need to know the future. As a product of the public educational system I always planned ahead, established goals, and expected results. The system had offered me a blueprint for life that told me if I followed the rules I would become a productive citizen. The system recommended that I get a degree or two, find a job, get married, pay taxes, and have a family. The school system also told me what to think and how to act. As a consequence of choosing to obey, I manifested dis-ease.

While the road to destiny is paved with good intentions, spirit has other plans. Spirit is the curious child, not afraid to buck the system. Spirit says be awkward and authentic. Be vulnerable and original. Be real and present. Speak openly and through the heart. And here's your opportunity for a chance to grow!

Awakening

With prescription in hand, it was time to question the face staring back at me in the mirror. Who was this woman other than mom, wife, daughter, sister, caregiver, chauffeur, and CEO (cook, educator, and organizer) of the home? If her life was so full, surrounded by people, why did she feel so alone? In her desire to grow up, create a family, and be responsible to others, had she neglected to be responsible to herself? Where had the happy girl with the imagination run off to?

For the next few months, feelings of despair, emptiness rose up uncontrolled as I released raw emotion. Tears flowed unpredictably. The dark and constricted areas were now open to the light.

During the day, I was acutely sensitive to energies in my environment and in other people. Indoors, I felt claustrophobic and needed to go outside to breathe. At times I felt ungrounded. When I described my situation to my sister, she suggested I begin a daily practice of meditation. So I began to meditate early in the morning, before the house woke up. In coming out of my head and into the silence of the heart, I unpacked all the baggage I'd brought with me—my stubbornness, my need to be right, my need to control my surroundings. I let go of the prevailing wisdom to allow the wisdom within to prevail. In this new space, and with a clear channel to spirit, I heard what my thyroid had been trying to tell me all along, if I had only listened to my body's language.

From the quietude, I opened to the message of my fifth chakra, which came to me as a knowing. What I knew is that in my attempt to play small, I had slammed shut the energetic doors of my voice and dimmed my light.

> CHAKRA—Sanskrit word meaning "wheel of light." The fifth chakra supplies universal energy, or *chi*, to the thyroid. This is Communications Central, equipped with inner podium and microphone and related to giving, receiving, and speaking truth.

Playing small is also about the third chakra. The third, solar plexus chakra of the gut is associated with personal power, will power, boundaries, and self-esteem. If unbalanced, it can swing between passivity and aggression. When balanced, it knows when to let go and when to take charge.

When one chakra is blocked there is inefficient flow of vital force through all the chakras. My light body, made up of mental, emotional, spiritual bodies, had known of my core deficiencies long before my physical symptoms ever appeared. Ego was the last to know and didn't take it well. But spirit reassured me that the message was delivered in divine time. And from this light of awareness came the true beginning of my healing journey.

In his book *Shaman, Healer, Sage*, Alberto Villoldo writes:

> The fifth chakra gives voice to the feelings of the heart. It speaks out of love, kindness, and forgiveness. In this center, the five elements—ether, earth, water, fire, air—are combined into pure energy. An awakened throat chakra brings us into the synchronicity with life.[54]

Especially since awakening is ongoing and never-ending. Meditation can help. But meditation practiced for the sake of *being* is not the answer. I am already *being* by being on Earth. Meditation allows you to focus inward to find wisdom to apply it in your relationships and interactions. Spending time in Nature is a form of meditation. Journaling to the steady sound of the waves or the music of the woods is a way to gain perspective on the energies entering your field to maintain your center and your sense of self. It can provide the space needed to upload your truth so you can act on it.

With focused attention in the heart, your higher energetic layers can inform and guide. According to the HeartMath Institute, the heart generates the largest electromagnetic field in the body.

HEART VS. BRAIN—The heart's electrical field, measured in an electrocardiogram is 60 times stronger than the brain and its magnetic field is 100 times stronger than the brain.

In the heart, we discover love as unconditional and without boundaries. We are able to better see our spiritual connection to ourselves, to each other, and to our surroundings. For me, the heart's location reflects a bridge between ego and spirit, a place of infinite love. It is Source energy, a direct connection to God, the divine. The heart chakra also contains the thymus gland, which is the neurological center of the immune system.

Our thoughts are generated from two base emotions, either love or fear. These psycho-emotional energies show up in the energy field weeks or months before they are observed in the physical body and can be visualized through the science of Kirlian photography. Using a special camera, each layer of the aura can be seen in living color, showing where holes and imbalances are located. We see how emotions are not abstract at all, and how a dominant thought over time causes imbalances in the body. After all, science tells us that emotions activate neuronal circuits to provoke biochemical reactions that change biology.

All disease begins when physical and emotional landscapes clash with our ability to balance our whole terrain. At a deeper level, disease begins with a lost connection to spirit. Every day that we wake up in the physical reality is a gift to express and grow our soul through our choices and actions. My body had sounded the alarm through its physical symptoms over many years, which I had chosen to ignore.

I knew that if I could understand the belief that caused me to become a victim of my own making then I might understand the broader epidemic of thyroid disease and how to reverse it in my body. The words of the authors I read continued to keep me company. They counseled me to step outside my protective box and go in the direction that pulled me. So after thirteen years of catering to my family's needs, I put one foot in front of the other to attend my first Health and Wellness conference put on by the Weston A. Price Foundation, which embraced traditional foods as medicine. Surrounded by the energy of a thousand like-minds, I felt as if I'd come home to my people.

SYNCHRONICITY

The energy at the conference, along with the food, energized me. I was drawn to an energy healer and I signed up for a thirty-minute private session. As I lay on his table, the healer's hands hovered over my body. He described a black tar-like gunk that clogged my uterus and an anger that congested my liver. As he moved the energy with his hands, he cleared subtle toxins from my colon to my heart. He suggested the herbal supplements of Hyssop for digestion and immune systems, and Hawthorn berries for the heart. After the session, he offered his assessment. He told me I absorb negative energy from others and should reinforce my boundaries by wrapping myself in a curtain of light each morning before beginning my day. He suggested honey to bring back the sweetness of life. I later learned that European herbalists believe the sweetness of honey added to hawthorn tea heals the heart. Before he was finished, he looked me in the eyes and said that I needed to look in the mirror and see myself as beautiful. He had seen completely through me. Though I was skeptical, I remained open-minded. In the spirit of 'believing is seeing,' I decided to trust the process.

Without too much thought to the session, I soon began to feel like a kid again, spontaneous, free, joyful. I felt lighter in my core. Throughout the rest of the conference, conversations flowed easily and instant connections were made. I did not want to leave the conference when it ended two days later.

What I didn't realize then was how the healing had sparked an opening between my subconscious and conscious minds. I began to notice synchronicities—signs of validation all around me. As I thought of certain people, there they were. As my perception shifted, I saw how synchronicities play into life on a daily basis, as they always had, if only I had been aware.

As I explored this new space, I slowly awoke to the awareness that the breakdown of my body's immune system had a deeper reality. The conference did more than connect me to like minds. A light had been switched on, showing me that I had been feeding a pattern of giving myself up for the sake of others, and of denying myself in my marriage over its nineteen years. The words of the energy healer resonated, showing me that in taking on other people's junk I had lost the joyful girl inside. As much as I had sought to make others comfortable and happy, I had neglected my own emotional needs. This revelation spoke to self-worth. When I returned home, the shadows awaited me.

Face-to-face with my reflection, I spoke my truth and voiced my needs. It was as if I'd picked up my spiritual shovel and unclogged the dam. In the process of releasing resistance, I had at least one answer as to why so many women have thyroid disease. With this new information, I had a choice: I could remain hostage to previous perceptions about myself or I could integrate the new information, be courageous, and change my pattern—and my biology along with it.

The curtain had been pulled back to reveal what I needed to see in order to begin the journey back home to myself. The message had been simply stated by the energy healer and I felt it in my bones. I needed to love myself.

> *Sometimes, it is easy to be generous outward, to give and give and give and yet remain ungenerous to yourself. You lose the balance of your soul if you do not learn to take care of yourself. You need to be generous to yourself in order to receive the love that surrounds you.*
>
> *— John O'Donohue, Anam Cara*

A few months later, my symptoms gone, I intuitively knew that my body no longer needed the natural thyroid hormone. During my first Health Freedom Expo in Chicago, I was again drawn to an energy healer who confirmed that my fifth chakra was clear. No thyroid dysfunction, so I stopped the hormone. Three months later, in a letter from my doctor, blood tests confirmed that my thyroid had returned to full function (see Appendix I).

I have read that if the fifth chakra is underactive, you will fail to express yourself and can be misunderstood or misinterpreted by others. If overactive, you are opinionated and may yell to get your point across. When the fifth chakra is balanced, you express yourself with ease and bring your creative ideas into manifestation on the physical level.

Rebalancing my thyroid also had consequences and casualties. It led to the end of my marriage. Yet no one was to blame. In shifting my view, I was simply no longer a match for my partner. Author Barbara Ann Brennan says the direction of growth happens through divine will. She writes:

> Divine will is a template of divine precision that is unfolding the perfect you. Will is not a force. The creative force of life is love. Divine precision creates an order in the universe that is outside of linear time.

Divine will comes from the soul. The soul is the driving force for growth, and soul growth is seen reflected at the level of the cell. Relationships between cells mirror the relationship with self. The relationship with self, in turn, mirrors our relationships with others.

The breakup of my marriage drew "a line in the sand" for me. It compelled me to step into a new awareness. My soul had been guiding me to stop lying to myself and express my authentic self. The only way she succeeded in getting my attention was through a complete shutdown of the gland that ran my entire body.

What you resist persists.
— Carl Jung, Swiss psychiatrist

By releasing resistance to my own voice, I allowed the vital force energy to run unimpeded. By being receptive, I slowly integrated more fully into my body. By forgiving myself, I gained confidence and value. I appreciated. Each new step became easier. I could offer my light without fear of having it diminished or extinguished. This light poured through me as I awoke to my inner calling. Taking a leap of faith in choosing the alternate path was not easy, but I can report that I landed on a bed of feathers.

> *The bad news is you're falling through the air, nothing to hang on to, no parachute. The good news is there's no ground.*
> — *Chögyam Trungpa Rinpoche, Buddhist Master*

THE POWER TO CHOOSE

An awareness that remains with me from my healing process is that the power to heal comes from the freedom to choose. My body my choice. Our choices give us free reign over the quality of our health and the dynamic of our relationships. I began to see how each relationship was a reflection of the relationship with myself and how the world mirrors to us the changes that we feel from within.

For example, when I worked as an environmental scientist for the U.S. Environmental Protection Agency I believed myself powerless to do anything to protect the air and water that lawmakers, officials, and the President seemed to ignore. I blamed others—politicians, corporations, the Agency where I worked—for postponing the mission to protect the health of the Earth and her people. In doing so, I took on the role of victim and failed to claim responsibility for my part. I went on to manifest an autoimmune disease. And I am not alone.

What appears to be the Earth coming apart at the seams—earth quaking, oil spewing, document leaking, stock market crashing, drug abusing, government corrupting, child molesting, liberty crushing, air polluting, industry controlling, disease exploding— is a pattern of the relationship with Self showing up for all of us, collectively.

Connecting these dots is to realize that the problem is reversible. If we don't like what we see around us, we only need to change our patterns to change the outcome. For me, it meant having the courage to shift my focus from my head to my heart and to see the beauty that was always there. Even if we cannot see the sun, it is always shining.

> *We are not physical beings having a spiritual experience; we are*
> *spiritual beings having a physical experience.*
> — *Pierre Teilhard de Chardin, French philosopher*

If we are each expressions of divinity, then there is no need to see anything but beauty and love when looking in the mirror. We existed in spiritual form before we were born into the physical world. First and foremost we are eternal Souls. What's not to love? We are connectors and transformers. We draw the people into life who help us and whom we help in return. The world is mirroring to us the changes we feel from within. If we understand this, we have the beginnings of a very empowering internal technology to reverse all disease.

The healing journey is a journey of choice. You can choose to see your diagnosis as a breakdown or a breakthrough. You can see yourself as a genetic defect or simply as out of balance. Your body has been responding exactly as it was designed to, with the tools you provided. Under Natural Law, you can access the tools of Nature so the body can reverse course. You can apply science along with wisdom. You have the ability to free your voice and find your own answers. A diagnosis, then, is an opportunity to step back and see the bigger picture, to accept this gift as the beginning of a journey into you, to take time to unwrap it, and to appreciate what it has to offer.

But I have gotten ahead of myself and sped to my own recovery. Let's back up. Most of us know someone with thyroid disease if we have not been diagnosed ourselves. The next steps in moving toward health are to ditch the label, discern the truth, and deconstruct the diagnosis. So what does the science say?

Ten Signs You Have An Underactive Thyroid:

- Fatigue after sleeping 8 to 10 hours a night or the need to take a nap daily.
- Weight gain or the inability to lose weight.
- Mood issues such as mood swings, anxiety, or depression.
- Hormone imbalances such as PMS, irregular periods, infertility, and low sex drive.
- Muscle pain, joint pain, carpal tunnel syndrome, or tendonitis.
- Cold hands and feet, feeling cold when others are not, or having a body temperature consistently below 98.5.
- Dry or cracking skin, brittle nails, and excessive hair loss.
- Constipation.
- Brain fog, poor concentration or poor memory.
- Neck swelling, snoring, or hoarse voice.

CHAPTER FIVE

DECONSTRUCT
THE DIAGNOSIS

KNOW YOUR THYROID

Your thyroid gland is a small butterfly-shaped organ located at the base of the throat, and the largest gland of the endocrine system. If your body is the Main Event, the thyroid it is the Master of Ceremonies, the master gland of metabolism. The basic unit of the thyroid gland is the follicle. Once the thyroid captures dietary iodine to produce thyroid hormone, thyroid hormone is stored in the center of the follicle until it is needed.

No gland functions in a void. Your thyroid works in concert with all your glands: the pineal, thalamus, hypothalamus and the pituitary glands, as well as the parathyroid glands, pancreas, kidneys, adrenals, thymus, ovaries, testes, and heart. They communicate by secreting specific messenger hormones that activate specific cell receptors. The thyroid's hormones influence every cell, tissue, and organ system in the body.[55] Thyroid hormones are not only created by the thyroid, but also by the ovaries, white blood cells, and bone marrow.

Your glands coordinate digestion, metabolism, oxygen consumption, heart rate and respiration, tissue function, sensory perception, sleep, excretion and detoxification, blood sugar regulation, energy, immune system, lactation, growth and development, movement, reproduction, mood, weight control, hair, skin, teeth, and nails, brain development and spiritual development so the body maintains balance.

WHAT MEDICAL CLASSIFICATION ARE YOU?

A medical label of thyroid disease means you are branded and further classified: *Hyperthyroidism, or Hypothyroidism* with subclassification: *mild, classical, profound.* You may also hear the words *progressive, permanent, and irreversible.* The doctor's voice rings in your ears as he tells you that, "your condition will require lifelong treatment since any abnormality of hormone synthesis can have far-reaching consequences on health."[56]

Did he say lifelong treatment? Did he say *abnormality*? Suddenly all those questions you were prepared to ask evaporate because the walls are closing in. The doctor proceeds to scribble some words on a white prescription pad, hands you the paper and says, "Here, this should help." And just like that, you find yourself corralled and branded. You've just joined the diseased and medicated herd.

Your diagnosis may overwhelm you, creating in you a sense of loss. You may feel small as your doctor reads off the results of your blood tests without taking a breath. His words run together in your head and make about as much sense to you as those of a mechanic who diagnoses that strange grinding noise from your car's engine.

You ask yourself how this could have happened. You have always been the picture of health and never experienced a weight problem before. You eat a healthy diet, to boot. You also exercise regularly and get enough rest, even though you've been unusually tired lately. So how did you get to this place? How did thyroid disease find *your* body?

DIAGNOSIS OF AN EPIDEMIC

Becoming diagnosed as part of the herd clearly means you are not alone. Today, thyroid disease is an epidemic that affects 59 million people in North America, four out of ten people, adults and children,[57] and more than 2.2 billion or 35 percent of the population worldwide.[58] Hypothyroidism is most common among women between the ages of 20 and 40.

Thyroid disease affects one out of five women and the number is rising. There is 9:1 greater prevalence in women than men. Eighty percent of thyroid disease is experienced by women with at least fifty percent of cases going undiagnosed.[59] Fifty-two percent of women diagnosed are under 50. The incidence of Hashimoto's thyroiditis is higher in women 40 years and older versus women 39 years and younger.[60]

One reason for a greater prevalence of thyroid disease in women is estrogen dominance. Estrogen and thyroid hormones have opposing actions. Too much estrogen blocks thyroid hormone from binding to its cell receptor and inhibits the absorption of iodine.[61] In addition, if you are a Type-O blood type, you are genetically prone to hypothyroidism and lower levels of iodine. Approximately 46 percent of people are blood Type-O.[62]

CLASSIFICATIONS AND SYMPTOMS

In the medical world, your diagnosis is based on the results of the 1960s-vintage blood test known as the Thyroid Stimulating Hormone (TSH) test. TSH is secreted by the pituitary and is, therefore, an indirect measure of thyroid function. If TSH levels are above a "normal" range, you are classified as Hypothyroid. If TSH levels fall below normal, you are classified as Hyperthyroid.

If diagnosed hypothyroid, Think Hippo. Your thyroid is underactive. Your energy is low. You make too little thyroid hormone. Metabolism slows down. With a sluggish thyroid you can experience symptoms of weight gain, sensitivity to cold and light due to low cellular energy, fatigue, digestive problems, constipation, high cholesterol, dry skin and hair, hair loss, fogginess, low libido, hoarse voice, muscle ache and weakness, joint pain, heavy periods, brittle nails/hair, depression, and irritability.

These days, who doesn't commiserate about one or more of these symptoms? There are at least three hundred known symptoms that describe a low functioning thyroid, many of which go undetected by blood tests. That is a lot of commiserating!

If diagnosed hyperthyroid, Think Hummingbird. Your thyroid is overactive. You make too much thyroid hormone. Metabolism speeds up. Excess hormones can pool in the blood which can lead to symptoms of weight loss, heat intolerance, excessive sweating, rapid heart rate, increased nervousness, diarrhea, irregular menstrual flow. There can be protuberant eyes (proptosis). Sufferers also experience fatigue, decreased concentration, and irritability.

About eighty percent of those diagnosed with thyroid disease are classified hypothyroid, while twenty percent are classified hyperthyroid. Eighty percent of those with hypothyroidism are autoimmune or "Hashimoto's." The 20 percent who are not autoimmune are likely heading in that direction as the body compensates and takes from its reserves to maintain homeostasis.

In autoimmune thyroiditis, the body creates antibodies against the thyroid, indicating inflammation (*itis*) and burning, which cause thyroid hormone production to swing. First, thyroid hormones leak out of the thyroid gland, raising hormone levels in the blood, leading to hyperthyroidism, which can last for one or two months before thyroid levels drop to reflect the hypothyroid state. This can happen postpartum due to fluctuating hormone levels.

Being diagnosed with profound hypothyroidism means you have some serious work ahead of you because your thyroid has completely burned out and shut down. The same condition is described in people whose thyroid has been removed. In this case you can experience extreme fatigue, shortness of breath, and swelling of the hands, face, feet, and tissues around the eyes, known as myxedema. Myxedema refers to the presence of a type of glycoprotein, mucin, found in almost all the connective tissues and organs of the body. Because thyroid hormone receptors are found on every cell membrane—in the interstitial fluid, the mitochondria and the nucleus—thyroid regulation is critical. The serious nature of this condition means your heart is at risk. Without immediate attention, this condition can lead to a coma and death.

IODINE, SELENIUM & HORMONES

The thyroid gland is a factory that requires the raw material, iodide. The iodide ion is the most abundant form of iodine on Earth, found in the oceans and the soil. Dietary iodide from food and water is absorbed from the gut into the blood, and then taken into the thyroid where it is concentrated and converted to organic iodine by the thyroid peroxidase enzyme. From here it is incorporated into tyrosine in a large glycoprotein thyroglobulin molecule within the thyroid follicular cell.[63] The digestion of thyroglobulin by lysosomal enzymes creates thyroid hormones thyroxine (T4) and triiodothyronine (T3) that are released into circulation. T4 can also be converted to T3 in target tissues such as the liver and brain by selenium-containing enzymes. This means selenium protects the thyroid during hormone synthesis. Any iodine left over is taken up by the extracellular fluids and excreted in the urine.

Iodine is vital. The diet provides only a small amount, 0.03 milligrams a day, or one-seventh of what is needed for daily hormone production. Fortunately, the body recycles much of the iodine stores and two-thirds of the iodine stores are located in the thyroid, which utilizes about 80μg iodine daily to synthesize hormones. Ninety percent of the hormone released by the thyroid is T4, which contains four iodine atoms. Without enough iodine, thyroid hormone production slumps, and results in thyroxine being stored in the gland rather than being released into circulation. This leads to engorgement of the gland, causing a goiter—a noticeable lump at the throat—as the thyroid attempts to ramp up production without the raw materials.

Historically, goiter was most common in populations that lacked sufficient iodine in the soil or water, or did not live near the ocean or eat a diet that included fish and seaweed, which contain iodine. Native Americans who lived away from the sea buried fish heads in their gardens to ensure a steady supply of iodine in their food. Today, goiter results from an inability to utilize iodine due to mercury toxicity from dental amalgams, and vaccines, and other toxic exposures.

MERCURY AND YOUR THYROID—Consider that 60-80 percent of the population has mercury fillings in their mouths and each filling releases 10 micrograms (µg) of mercury vapor daily into lungs and saliva. Mercury released from a gold alloy bridge amounts to 30 µg per day. These levels far exceed government health standards of 1 µg/day for the 'average' adult.64 Amalgam exposure alone, is reason enough for the body to select for more reverse T3 to slow itself down.

Mercury affects the four small parathyroid glands in back of the thyroid. The parathyroid produces parathyroid hormone to regulate blood-calcium levels, as well as phosphorous and vitamin D metabolism. As the thyroid requires iodine, the parathyroids require boron.

Mercury also accumulates in the adrenal glands to disrupt gland function. During stress, the adrenals increase in size as a normal reaction in order to produce more steroid hormones. Mercury also builds in the pituitary gland and depletes the adrenals of both pantothenic acid and vitamin C. Therefore, stress and the presence of mercury have a combined negative impact on the adrenals and the production of critical hormones.

Conversion of T4 Thyroid Hormone

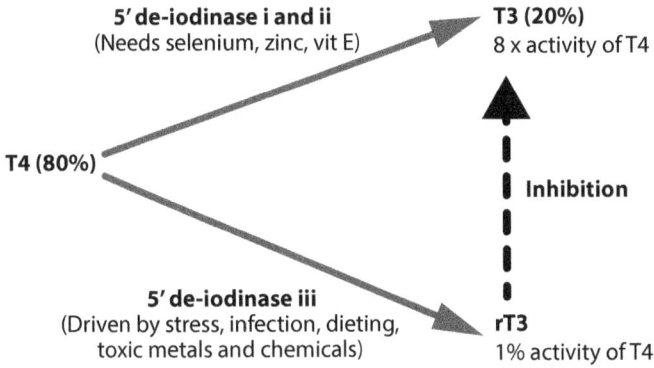

5' de-iodinase i and ii
(Needs selenium, zinc, vit E)

T3 (20%)
8 x activity of T4

T4 (80%)

Inhibition

5' de-iodinase iii
(Driven by stress, infection, dieting,
toxic metals and chemicals)

rT3
1% activity of T4

Figure No. 2

When T4 hormone is released from the thyroid, it circulates throughout the body and converts a portion of itself into two metabolites that are mirror images of each other: Forty percent becomes T3 (triiodothyronine) and twenty percent becomes reverse T3 (rT3) in the liver and kidneys.

T3 is the bioactive form of thyroid hormone due to its stronger affinity for thyroid receptors. When T3 binds to cells, it up-regulates cell metabolism. When rT3 binds to cells, it down-regulates cell metabolism. Signals from the body's terrain determine which form binds to cell receptors.

The conversion of T4 to T3 is critical. Conversion not only requires iodine and its enzyme, but also fat-soluble vitamins A and D, as well as selenium, zinc, iron, copper, manganese, molybdenum vitamin D3, vitamin E, L-tyrosine, and vitamin B2, B3, B6, B12 in their methylated form.

It is always best to get nutrients through Nature. Organic kelp provides a ready source of iodine and co-nutrients. One-quarter cup of dried seaweed may contain as much as 4500 µg iodine, though any amount above 1100 µg cannot be legally recommended based on the U.S. RDA guideline for iodine. Guggul gum (*Commiphora mukul),* a resin from a thorny tree that grows in India, is used in Ayurvedic medicine to promote the conversion of T4 to T3 hormone. Myrrh extract, an essential oil, is similar to guggul, and along with myrtle essential oil, supports thyroid hormone conversion. Thyroid glandulars also improve the conversion of T4 to T3.

Factors that block T4-T3 conversion and its enzyme at the level of the cell include stress, weight gain, obesity, infection, trauma, depression, radiation, medications, exposure to toxins and plastics, pesticides, mercury, metals, autoimmune disease, diabetes, insulin resistance, and liver and kidney dysfunction. These are the same factors that preferentially select for the inactive form—rT3—to bind at the cell.

STRESS AND LOW STOMACH ACID

The one thing that trumps a healthy diet and lifestyle is stress, which makes stress 100 percent the cause of disease. In times of stress, the body is designed to hibernate. Reverse T3 is the "hibernation hormone." It binds to cell receptors to down-regulate metabolism, to slow you down, so you are forced to rest. During stress, the enzyme which converts T4 to T3 is suppressed. One job of rT3 is to clear excess T4 so it doesn't pool in the blood. At rT3 levels greater than 50 percent (>150), there is a need to address inflammation. High rT3 is an indicator of either: 1) iron deficiency, 2) copper deficiency 3) cortisol imbalance, or 4) a combination of these. Inflammation can mean poor digestion and low stomach acid.

Many symptoms of hypothyroidism are the same symptoms of low stomach acid. Low stomach acid leads to decreased red blood cells and anemia. Low stomach acid results in ineffective break down of protein in the stomach. Large proteins migrate to the small intestine and cause stress to the pancreas. If "leaky gut" exists, proteins leak into the blood to cause the body to create antibodies and autoimmunity. As pH shifts, microbes shift to Candida and parasites. Low stomach acid also decreases the absorption of thyroid hormone by 25 percent, which can lead to hypothyroidism[65] and may require an increase of thyroid hormone dose by 25 percent. Supplementing with proteolytic enzymes improves stomach acid production, promotes protein digestion, and cleans the blood to optimize blood flow. Herbal bitters do the same. Herbal formulations include orange peel, ginger root, gentian root, peppermint leaf, goldenseal root, hops flower, cardamom seed, fennel seed, Oregon grape root, blessed thistle herb, hawthorn, cayenne pepper, burdock root and dandelion root.

FACTORS THAT AFFECT THYROID FUNCTION

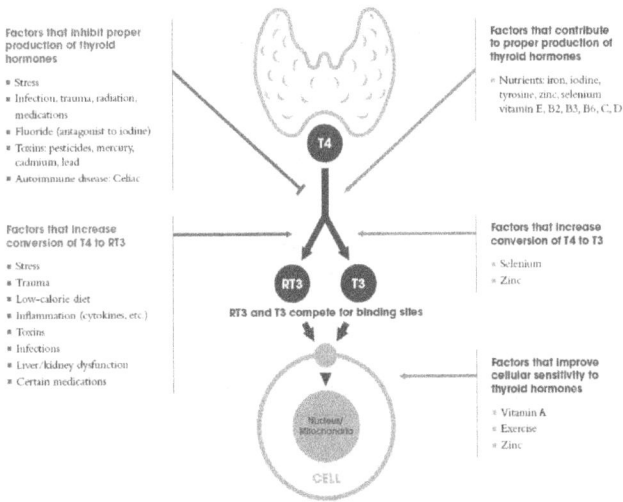

Factors that inhibit proper production of thyroid hormones

- Stress
- Infection, trauma, radiation, medications
- Fluoride (antagonist to iodine)
- Toxins: pesticides, mercury, cadmium, lead
- Autoimmune disease: Celiac

Factors that contribute to proper production of thyroid hormones

- Nutrients: iron, iodine, tyrosine, zinc, selenium vitamin E, B2, B3, B6, C, D

Factors that increase conversion of T4 to RT3

- Stress
- Trauma
- Low-calorie diet
- Inflammation (cytokines, etc.)
- Toxins
- Infections
- Liver/kidney dysfunction
- Certain medications

Factors that increase conversion of T4 to T3

- Selenium
- Zinc

RT3 and T3 compete for binding sites

Factors that improve cellular sensitivity to thyroid hormones

- Vitamin A
- Exercise
- Zinc

T4 RT3 T3 Nucleus/Mitochondria CELL

Figure No. 3

The ability to synthesize thyroid hormone from iodine is retained by each cell. This was discovered in tadpole experiments that showed that when the thyroid was removed and iodine given in any form, metamorphosis continued at the same rate, as if thyroid hormone was present. In humans, thyroid disease symptoms begin when thyroid hormone levels decline inside each cell.

All the glands are communicating with each other to keep the energy moving. The brain's hypothalamus picks up this signal and sends its messenger hormone TSH (Thyroid Stimulating Hormone) to the pituitary to tell the thyroid to increase production. In response, the thyroid releases more T4, T3 and rT3 hormones to all cells, and reports back (in a negative feedback loop) to the hypothalamus and pituitary.

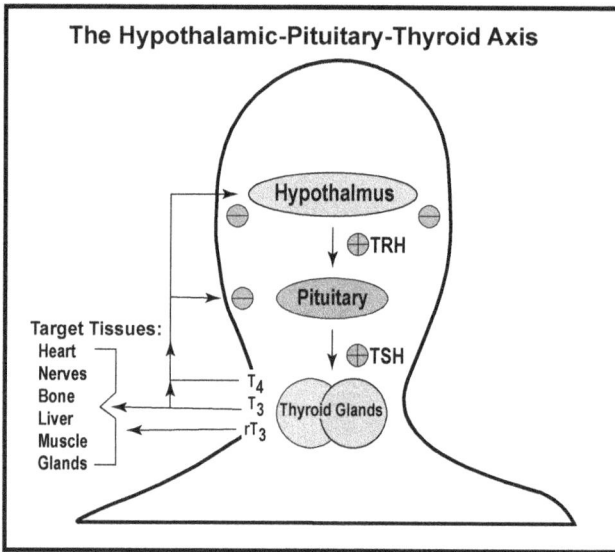

Figure No. 4

ARE YOU DEFECTIVE?

The body is self-regulating and does the best it can given the tools it has to use. The universal Law of Cause and Effect says that for every effect there is a cause. However, your physician will diagnose and treat thyroid disease without identifying a cause, except to offer up one or more of the following reasons for thyroid dysfunction... if you ask:

- It's the thyroid's fault—that is, it produces too little or too much hormone.
- It's a genetic defect, failure to methylate—that is, your genetic make-up, nothing to do about *that*.
- It's Idiopathic—that is, we don't know.

After six to eight years of medical school and residency, the best explanation your physician can provide about your condition is that it is caused by your genes. A diagnosis means you can blame your parents while the doctor is off the hook. Because his cognitive bias is based on his training, his treatment options fall under the law of the hammer, where everything looks like a nail. But you can carefully choose the tools you work with when it comes to your body.

It is important to be skeptical of any official opinion that claims to hold the key to your genetic signature since you are a metaphysical being living in a physical body. You are more than your reflection in the mirror or a series of numbers from a blood test taken at one point in time.

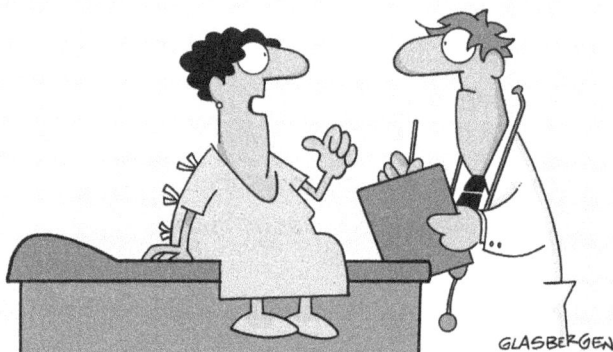

"You have to learn about thousands of diseases, but
I only have to focus on fixing what's wrong with ME!
Now which one of us do you think is the expert?"

*Science cannot solve the ultimate mystery of nature. And that
is because, in the last analysis, we ourselves are a part of the
mystery that we are trying to solve.*

— *Max Planck, Where Is Science Going?*

While your genetics may predispose you to certain weaknesses and patterns, genes do not determine outcome. Genes are blueprints. They can only execute their instructions when triggered by signals in the environment or by other cells. Your genes are enhanced or diminished according to your experiences and the choices you make, including what you eat whether you smoke, and if you exercise. How you live your life determines the quality of your genes and what you pass onto future generations, both physically and energetically. That goes beyond genetics to epigenetics, which will be explored further in chapter eight.

A diagnosis becomes an opportunity for introspection. When you have a diagnosis of thyroid disease, you have some choices to make. There is no right or wrong answer. There is only your answer.

Doing nothing is a choice; however, if ignored, thyroid disease can progress to heart disease, infertility, osteoporosis, thyroid cancer, coma, and death.[66]

Always deconstruct the diagnosis. You are not a disease label or a genetic defect. In order to discern the truth about who you are, get to know your True Self on an intimate level. If you know what you hunger for, you're one step closer to the cause of imbalance. When you identify the cause then you are one step closer to the cure.

CHAPTER SIX

TRUTH ABOUT
TREATMENTS AND TESTING

Licensed medical doctors are the only doctors authorized to "prescribe," "treat," and "diagnose" disease conditions. These doctors practice licensed medicine because the dangers of their FDA-approved treatments can come with adverse side effects, black box warnings, and an LD50; the lethal dose of a drug that kills 50 percent of the population tested.

ALLOPATHIC TREATMENTS
Allopathic medicine offers a one-size-fits-all synthetic thyroid hormone, levothyroxine known as Synthroid to improve thyroid function. Synthroid contains a small amount of iodine but not enough to restore thyroid function. Also included in the drug's formula are acacia, confectioner's sugar, D&C Yellow No. 10, FD&C Blue No. 1, FD&C Yellow No. 6, lactose, magnesium stearate, povidone, and talc, a known carcinogen.

If you consent to this T4-only drug, you will be required to retest your blood every six months for the rest of your life to ensure a stable dose-response relationship based on a range of "average" values. Your blood-sacrifice does not indicate a deficiency of Synthroid, so expect symptoms to continue while on the drug. Synthroid will not balance mineral deficiencies or a lack of communication between the endocrine glands, nor will it address any physiological and emotional imbalances. Make room in your schedule for extra visits to adjust the dose when the drug fails to make you feel better. This is why you are called *patient*.

If you are a poor T4 converter, then T3 hormone will not meet its target cells. If you are over-medicated with T4, you may develop hyperthyroid symptoms of tachycardia, insomnia, and anxiety. Drug potency is not guaranteed since Synthroid is unstable in the presence of light, temperature, air, and humidity. Due to its instability, Synthroid has been the subject of court disputes based on numerous recalls for failure to meet potency. [67]

According to the package insert, Synthroid is contraindicated in patients with uncorrected adrenal insufficiency. Synthroid may worsen glycemic control in patients with diabetes mellitus and may result in increased insulin requirements. Decreased bone mineral density may occur. Those with coronary artery disease and cardiovascular disease should watch for increased symptoms of coronary insufficiency and be monitored closely if taking Synthroid. Adverse reactions mimic hyperthyroidism as arrhythmias, myocardial infarction, dyspnea, muscle spasm, headache, nervousness, irritability, insomnia, tremors, muscle weakness, increased appetite, weight loss, diarrhea, heart intolerance, menstrual irregularities, and skin rash.

Over time, your body will recognize Synthroid as a toxin because Synthroid's chemicals create a congested liver. A congested liver cannot filter the blood or transform food. Backed-up toxins are eliminated through the skin resulting in skin rashes. Unassimilated protein produces poisons which invade the blood, intestines, and kidneys. Both the liver and kidneys contribute to the acid-base equilibrium of blood pH. If the acid level is high, the kidneys eliminate excess through the urine. If liquids are not eliminated due to kidney congestion, they stagnate in the tissues and cause swelling, uric acid, oxalic acid, lactic acid and salts, which negatively impacts the central nervous system and nerves throughout the body.

Excess toxins lead to a shift in pH which leads to a shift of our beneficial microbes. When metabolic pathways are thrown off, the body cannot efficiently eliminate toxins, which leads to systemic inflammation and adrenal exhaustion. As your body's resistance builds against the drug, the drug loses effectiveness.

Over time, your doctor can offer no solutions other than to adjust the dose of a hormone that is fast losing value. Doctors will not suggest cleansing a congested liver or kidneys or detoxing other organs such as the colon, gallbladder, kidneys, blood, and lymph glands to bring thyroid function back. They will not suggest changing your diet to include more organic fruits and vegetables to cleanse the blood. Thousands of years earlier, the ancient Egyptians, Chinese, Babylonians, and Greeks made the enema a part of normal cleansing hygiene. The Egyptians of 1500 BC utilized coffee enemas three days each month. For millennia, the Pharaohs had a "guardian of the anus," a doctor who administered the royal enema.

Synthetic Vs. Natural Hormones

Hormones work together within the body's self-regulating system to maintain homeostasis. One problem with adding a synthetic, T4-only treatment is that your body naturally makes at least five different thyroid hormones, such as T4, T3, rT3 T2, T1, each with its own special function. Alternatives to Synthroid include natural dessicated thyroid hormones that are either porcine-derived or yam-derived. However, you must be ready to suggest one of these alternative therapies since your physician will not offer it as an option.

While doctors can legally suggest bio-identical hormones from a compounding pharmacy, they face intimidation by FDA officials in doing so. Federal authorities criminalize physicians who suggest natural remedies as a felony under "fraudulent billing" through the systems of Medicare, Medicaid, and the Veterans Administration, and as a condition of their employment, backed up by Medical Board Regulations.[68]

Your doctor may suggest a combination T4-T3 therapy of Levothyroxine and Liothyronine if T4-only Levothyroxine therapy fails to work. However, several published studies report there is no obvious benefit over T4-only therapy.[69] [70] Two double-blind, randomized, controlled trials failed to show any improvement in depressive symptoms[71] or fatigue[72] in those with hypothyroidism.

When T4-T3 therapies fail, a T3-only therapy may be suggested (if T3/rT3 <20). However, be aware that the direct negative effects include dementia, hair loss, muscle wasting, and bone loss—all severe symptoms of hypothyroidism. Further, excess T3 can trigger high inactive rT3 hormone to cause imbalances in other hormones. Since no continuous real-time testing of T4-T3 ratios is ever performed, the outcome of synthetic hormone dosing is ineffectual.

IS RADIATION THERAPY A GOOD IDEA?

Radioactive iodine, as radioiodine, is one of three standard medical treatments for Graves' disease, including antithyroid drugs and thyroidectomy. Radioiodide is known to induce hypothyroidism in 90 percent of patients within the first year, with a continuing rate of 2-3 percent per year thereafter.[73]

Radioiodide is only effective if your aim is to destroy the thyroid gland because you believe the cause of the problem is excessive thyroid tissue. This radioactive isotope, known as I-131, will destroy surrounding cells wherever it binds. Its use has been linked to leukemia and other forms of cancer.[74] The list of symptoms sounds like a TV drug advertisement: Fifteen percent of patients are on anti-thyroid drugs, or goitrogens. They report fever and arthralgia[75] and may be more prone to infections. Goitrogens can induce severe liver toxicity, requiring liver transplantation, sometimes resulting in death.[76]

Based on his success in reversing thyroid disease using iodine therapy, Dr. Guy E. Abraham writes:

> Indeed, we have a zombified medical profession. Case in point, patients are told to protect their thyroid gland from radioactive fallout by ingesting inorganic iodine [then] if diagnosed with Graves' disease, are told to stop taking inorganic, non-radioactive iodine/iodide to penetrate their thyroid gland. Does that make any sense?[77]

Human studies after the 1986 Chernobyl nuclear disaster show examples of the health consequences experienced by a large population, especially children, exposed to radioactive iodine.[78] Children who were younger than 10 at the time of the disaster showed that ionizing radiation induces a type of DNA damage known as fusion oncogenes that form papillary thyroid cancer a quarter century later.[79]

The consequences of the nuclear disaster at Fukushima in 2011 have not been fully determined since papillary thyroid cancer develops at a slow pace. In humans, cancers associated with radiation exposure are mostly papillary carcinoma, while those associated with iodine-deficient areas are more often follicular.[80] [81]

This point is worth repeating. Radiation causes cancer. Radiation is used to induce cancer in lab rats.[82] Radioactive therapy prior to bone marrow transplants as a treatment for Hodgkin's disease is a major risk factor for subsequent thyroid cancer and removal of the thyroid.[83] In evaluating thyroid cysts in children, ultrasound has proven more useful than laboratory tests and less harmful than radionuclide testing.[84] [85] There are always natural alternatives to investigate before turning to radiation.

NATURAL REMEDIES

In cases of emergency radiation exposures, such as in Chernobyl, potassium iodide (KI) reduces levels of radioactive iodine uptake by the thyroid to prevent later development of thyroid cancer.[86] *Not more radiation.* The thyroid absorbs both stable and radioactive iodine and cannot distinguish the difference. Potassium iodide is a salt of stable iodine used as medicine. KI comes in both liquid and tablet forms. Iodine only protects the thyroid from radiation, not other parts of the body. When the thyroid becomes "full," it is unable to absorb more iodine—either stable or radioactive—for the next 24 hours.

Many natural remedies exist that prove successful in reversing a radiation body burdens. Post-Chernobyl, apple pectin was used to reduce Cesium-137 levels by up to 60 percent[87] in as few as 16 days[88] in exposed children. Apple pectin also prevents Plutonium-239 from being absorbed in the intestine.[89] Phytochemicals in apples are responsible for pulling out metals and radiation. Other detox protocols include chlorella, amino acid glutamine, sea vegetables, Atlantic kelp and dulse, lemon water (half a lemon squeezed in a 16-oz glass on empty stomach upon awakening), and green juice fasting. Example homeopathic remedies against the direct negative effects of radiotherapy include *Ruta Graveolens, Nux Vomica, Fluoricum Acidum, and X-ray*. Consult a homeopath for the right remedy and dosing.

Bentonite clay was dumped into Chernobyl's nuclear reactors after the nuclear meltdown. Russian scientists are known to coat their bodies with bentonite clay for protection when working with radiation. The ingestion of small amounts of bentonite clay can be used internally and immediately and should be accompanied by clay baths from twenty minutes to one hour, as individuals tolerate. Twenty-minute clay compresses applied to target the lymphatic system and primary organs can also be used.

NATURAL THYROID THERAPIES

In choosing a temporary treatment to balance hormones, natural thyroid hormone preparations are recommended. Natural hormones made to standards approved by the United States Pharmacopeia assure an accurate potency as stated on the label. The most popular brands include Armour Thyroid, Westhroid, Nature Thyroid, and a bio-identical compounded formulation made from yam available at the Women's International Pharmacy.

Iodine researcher and developer of an iodine assay, Dr. Guy Abraham, believes thyroid hormones are an expensive form of the element iodine, which is what patients really need based on the self-evident fact that the whole body, not just the thyroid gland, needs iodine. Iodine plays different roles in different organs and tissues. Holistic doctors who understand the body's need for both iodine and iodide utilize inorganic, non-radioactive iodine/iodide in the form of Lugol's iodine, and other forms.[90]

IODINE AND MAGNESIUM SUPPLEMENTATION

Iodine supplementation regulates immune function by not only creating thyroid hormones, but also through shifting the conditions of the terrain so the microbiome returns to homeostasis. Iodine is a natural anti-microbial and also detoxifies the body through increased urinary excretion of lead, cadmium, arsenic, aluminum, and mercury. Iodine in the form of Kelp, dulse, detoxified iodine, Nascent iodine, Lugol's iodine, or Iosol, a patented low-dose formula, benefits the thyroid naturally.

Because magnesium deficiency is pervasive in the population, Dr. Guy E. Abraham suggests a safe nutritional treatment using iodine and magnesium together, of which magnesium intake is between 800-1,200 mg daily. This type of nutritional approach is important in the reversal of both Hashimoto's disease and Graves' autoimmune thyroiditis."[91]

HOMEOPATHIC REMEDIES

For those worried about whether or not elemental iodine can cause thyroid pathology, homeopathic iodum or bromium or thyroidinum, or others, might be considered as energetic remedies to antidote the specific symptoms of imbalance. The chosen remedy and dose is always specific to the person and totality of symptoms: person-specific, not disease-specific. Therefore, remedies are best chosen by a trained homeopathic doctor.

GLANDULARS

Glandular therapy can be an alternate therapy to thyroid hormones. Thyroid glandulars use animal tissues to enhance the function of the corresponding human tissue based on the law of similars, or "like cures like," and because glands offer biologically active substances normally secreted by the gland. Most glandular products come from bovine sources, except for pancreatic glandulars, which come from pigs. Glands are prepared using either freeze-drying, or predigestion, which use plant or animal enzymes to hydrolyze the material. It is important that the glands derive from organically raised, grass-fed, healthy animals from open ranges. Adrenal glandular supplementation may also be considered. A naturopath can help determine if one or both glands need support and if other mineral deficiencies need to be addressed.

THE TRUTH ABOUT TESTING

There are three main reasons why at least fifty percent of people with thyroid conditions go undetected. First, "normal" for a lab test is based upon 2.5 standard deviations of those tested. Therefore, there is no truly representative "healthy range" since the pool is taken as an average sample. The same is true for veterinary labs that perform thyroid tests on animals that lump together every dog and cat to develop norms and averages.[92]

Secondly, the diagnostic blood tests of thyroid hormones are problematic since they are not sensitive enough to detect milder forms of hypothyroidism. The TSH test, developed in the 1960s, is used exclusively as the "gold standard" as part of the pituitary feed back loop to monitor the thyroid gland. If the TSH level is above the normal range, a patient is diagnosed as hypothyroid; TSH levels below normal range are interpreted as hyperthyroidism.

Remember, TSH levels fluctuate to reflect the needs of the pituitary gland.[93] TSH represents only the brain's need for thyroid hormone because thyroid metabolism is controlled locally in the tissues of each organ. A study of thyroid disease prevalence found that sixty percent of patients taking thyroid hormone continue to have abnormal thyroid function and forty percent of patients who took thyroid medications had abnormal TSH levels.[94] Further, TSH measurements can lag years behind symptoms, and because the numbers can fluctuate widely, such testing does not reflect actual thyroid function.[95]

TSH alone does not indicate whether you are creating antibodies against your thyroid (autoimmune thyroiditis), or whether you have an underlying adrenal problem, low stomach acid, or any number of physical conditions related to thyroid insufficiency. This test also does not address the underlying cause, which is inflammation.

A typical thyroid panel usually includes a thyroxine (T4) blood test, which accounts for ninety percent of the hormone secretion by the thyroid. However, you now know that if you cannot convert T4 to the bioactive T3 form then you do not know what is happening at the level of the cell. Someone with "normal levels" of T4 could be thyroid-deficient.

The best medical blood test for thyroid inflammation, according to a 2005 study in the *Journal of Clinical Endocrinology*

& Metabolism is the ratio of free T3/rT3 ratio. This ratio *is the most useful marker for hypothyroidism at the level of the cell.*[96] RT3 can also be obtained by subtracting free T3 from total T3 as long as units are the same. With the free T3/rT3 ratio, healthy ratios will be 20 or higher. With a total T3/rT3 ratio, you are looking for 10 units or higher where the units are the same.

David Derry M.D., Ph.D., a thyroid expert and biochemistry researcher, believes that the TSH test has no correlation to clinical presentation, except when symptoms are extreme, because it is unrelated to how the patient feels. According to Dr. Derry, there are many mechanisms by which each tissue controls the amount of thyroid hormone that gets into the tissues but the main elements are special enzymes, the deiodinases, which take one iodine atom off the thyroxine T4 to make T3 or triiodothyronine.[97] Imbalances in the nervous system, endocrine system, immune system, metabolism, and nutritional status can *all* affect thyroid signaling.[98] Therefore, it is important to note your symptoms and check for toxicities and deficiencies.

BEST TEST FOR THYROID FUNCTION

The best indicator of thyroid function is the Iodine loading test. This 24-hour test represents the previous day's dietary iodine intake, as over ninety percent of iodine absorbed is eventually excreted in the urine. Values below 50 µg/liter are abnormal. According to Dr. Hakala, a simple urine test he developed could confirm a faulty iodine transport system. To order a test kit, contact Hakala Labs online.

EVALUATE ANEMIA: IRON, COPPER, AND ZINC

Thyroid evaluation should also include checking iron, copper, and zinc blood levels. Anemia is common in both hypothyroidism and hyperthyroidism. It is often associated with an iron deficiency and treated with iron supplementation. However, anemia can reflect an imbalance in the ratio between iron, copper, and zinc. These three elements all work together in preventing and correcting thyroid disease. If any one of them is out of balance, it can deplete the other two. For instance, if zinc goes up, copper and iron go down. High doses of iron can create a copper deficiency and worsen anemia, as well as constipation. [99]

An iron deficiency may mean iron is locked up in tissues due to not enough bioavailable copper. Increasing copper intake through foods such as organ meats, especially liver, leafy greens, cocoa, beans, bee pollen, potatoes, and prunes can release iron stored in the liver, heart, and endocrine system, to make it available for red blood cell formation. Copper is essential for elastin in tissue, which keeps everything pliable. It is also an antiviral, anti-parasite, anti-fungal, anti-tumor, and anti-inflammatory, strengthens blood and clears arteries, protects against strokes and convulsive seizures, supports the CNS and brain cells, and supports a healthy immune system.

Anemia can also reflect low stomach acid from mineral imbalances, which can decrease the absorption of thyroid hormone by 25 percent.[100] Low stomach acid changes the species of bacteria present in the stomach to undesirable forms. It also results in ineffective breakdown of protein in the stomach, which allows large proteins to migrate to the small intestine and cause stress to the pancreas. Large proteins combined with leaky gut means proteins leak into the blood to cause the body to create antibodies and autoimmunity. This process fuels bacterial overgrowth, Candida (yeast) and parasites as pH shifts in the tissues.

A medical doctor may prescribe antacid drugs, which further lower the absorption through the gut wall and slow metabolism, exacerbating hypothyroidism.[101] Alternatively, supplementing with Betaine HCL and proteolytic enzymes improves stomach acid production and protein digestion. Herbal bitters also support the digestive system and acid production. Depending on the individual, formulations can include orange peel, ginger root, gentian root, peppermint leaf, goldenseal root, hops flower, cardamom seed, fennel seed, Oregon grape root, blessed thistle herb, hawthorn, cayenne pepper, burdock root and dandelion root.

EPIDEMIC OF FALSE CLAIMS AND CONFLICTS OF INTEREST

A sobering analysis of studies published in the prestigious 2013 *New England Journal of Medicine* found that forty percent—146 practices of current screening tests, diagnostic tests, medical procedures, medication, and surgery—showed no benefit. Findings were reversed, meaning they never worked in the first place based on faulty data.[102]

Marcia Angell, former Editor-in-Chief at the *New England Journal of Medicine*, wrote a 2009 article called "Drug Companies & Doctors: A Story of Corruption" where she claimed: [103]

> It is simply no longer possible to believe much of the clinical research that is published, or to rely on the judgment of trusted physicians or authoritative medical guidelines. I take no pleasure in this conclusion, which I reached slowly and reluctantly over my two decades as an editor of *The New England Journal of Medicine*.

Stanford statistician John Ioannidis exposed the widespread problem of fraudulent claims in his 2005 paper in *PLOS Medicine* stating, "most current published research findings are false."[104] In a 2001 *Scientific American* article, he reported:

> False positives and exaggerated results in peer-reviewed scientific studies have reached epidemic proportions in recent years. The problem is rampant in economics, the social sciences and even the natural sciences, but it is particularly egregious in biomedicine.[105]

Over the last 35 years, thousands of studies have come under scrutiny based on estimates that 20 to 36 percent of cell lines scientists use are contaminated or misidentified as human cells when they originate from pigs, rats, mice, or tainted human cells. One tainted human cell line is the HeLa cell line of cancerous cervical cells taken from 31-year-old, African-American Henrietta Lacks, first cultured in the 1950s without her permission. These cells are ubiquitous in labs, proliferate uncontrolled, and contaminate all cell lines in which they come into contact.[106]

> *We're looking at tens of thousands of publications, millions of journal citations, and potentially hundreds of millions of research dollars."*[107]
>
> — *Christopher Korch, geneticist*

Science and ethics part ways when deception is published as fact. Large pharmaceutical companies have also been caught creating their own fake peer-reviewed medical journals to convince doctors and the public that phony data is favorable.[108] Naturally, we must question the contradiction of a rising prevalence of autoimmune disease under a narrative of "the world's most advanced medical system." Blatant conflicts of interest and fraud show that mainstream medicine places profit over accountability and disease management over health care. The true nature of our bodies has been known by many cultures for over tens of thousands of years. Our answers are found within, and therefore, are within reach for each of us.

CHAPTER SEVEN

IODINE AND THE THYROID

Thyroid disease is Iodine Deficiency Disease. Indeed, modern medicine was founded on evidence that goiter, which is an enlarged thyroid gland and a specific disorder, could be reversed by iodine, a specific mineral. Allopathic medicine did not begin as chemical, but nutritional, based on the understanding that every cell in the body requires iodine. Known as "The Metabolizer," iodine was prescribed and utilized for more than 180 years as an essential nutrient, not a drug.

Historically, iodine was not only used to treat goiter and hypothyroidism, but also used to help reverse dermatologic conditions, chronic lung disease, fungal infestations, tertiary syphilis, and even arteriosclerosis. Iodine had been the universal choice of doctors who considered it a panacea for all ills due to its broad medicinal effects. Once upon a time, doctors observed that symptoms of iodine deficiency mirror symptoms of hypothyroidism: poor circulation, high homocysteine levels, low blood pressure, high cholesterol, low libido, weight gain/loss, lack of appetite, bloating, fluid retention, constipation, liver and kidney conditions, [109] skin problems, dry eyes, cataracts, aching joints, sensitivity to cold, graying hair, and hair loss.[110] History also shows that without enough iodine, mental retardation, abnormal gait, and short stature also result.

Even in light of irrefutable evidence, iodine remains relatively unknown as a preventative and disease reversal tool because it is not a patentable product for the profit-driven pharmaceutical industry that subsidizes the medical schools. Moreover, the sale of iodine in the form of Lugol's iodine, a mixture of iodine and potassium iodide, has largely been criminalized and outlawed.

To attempt to outlaw nature is futile and absurd when large amounts of the trace mineral, iodine, are found in the breast, skin, stomach, salivary glands, brain, pancreas, thymus, skin, and more than half the body's immune system. Iodine even helps you sweat. Iodine not only makes thyroid hormones, but also manufactures all other hormones.

Since you must get iodine from your food, you can find it in seaweed, cod liver oil, organic dairy, seafood, eggs, and organ meats. Today, however, most people do not live near the sea or have access to a fresh supply of wild caught, clean fish or sea vegetables. Iodine is transported into cells via the sodium-iodine (NIS) symporter.

The NIS is an ion pump that carries iodide into thyroid epithelium cells. Iodine studies by Drs. Jorge Flechas and Guy Abraham found that in some cases, no matter how much iodine people consumed they would not become iodine sufficient if the body's NIS had become dysfunctional due to a genetic defect. Even when iodine is absorbed into the GI tract from food, iodine does not always get into the cells. This may also be due to an inefficient oxidation of intracellular iodide.[111] Oxidation requires a steady supply of oxygen flowing through the interstitial tissues for cell oxygen uptake.

OXYGEN, pH, AND IODINE

The common symptoms of hypothyroidism—fatigue, cold-intolerance, infertility, and hair loss—reflect reduced cell oxygen uptake. Oxygen is directly influenced by pH; the more alkaline the tissues, the more the interstitial fluids can hold oxygen for the cells. Where oxygen is the fuel, iodine is the match that lights the flame of metabolism. When thyroid hormones decline due to lack of iodine, the body cannot convert food to energy. The thyroid does not get access to iodine unless body pH is optimal. Iodine also requires an optimal pH in order to be assimilated.[112]

The pH of an ecosystem is a measure of oxygen, and cell voltage. When cells become acidic, they dump alkaline waste into the blood. This waste blocks energy flow and causes ideal blood pH to rise to 7.5 or higher, making an ideal home for mold—cancer—to thrive. Because cancer will die at a blood pH of 7.35 or lower, the way to heal is to reverse the process. Increasing cell nutrition—minerals—increases pH in the cells, increases oxygen throughput, increases voltage, and brings the cells back into balance.

Iodine is an adaptogen. It gives the body what it needs to stabilize pH. It pulls minerals from tissues such as sodium, potassium, calcium, and magnesium to neutralize acids. Iodine increases metabolism and oxygen delivery to cells. Oxygen buffers metabolic waste acids to create a more alkaline pH. When pH and oxygen improve, so does cell voltage. Thus, supplying iodine, while also adding magnesium and selenium for the immune system, increases oxygen and voltage to increase cell energy and shift the microbes to beneficial forms.[113] The disease process is not linear but electrodynamic with the whole system moving in harmonic resonance based on the inherent healing ability of each individual's terrain.

How Much Iodine?

The human body can hold 1500 mg of iodine, of which the thyroid holds a maximum of 50 mg. In general, the body's daily requirements of iodine are 6 mg/day for the thyroid, 5 mg/day for the breasts, and 2 mg/day for your other glands such as your adrenals, pituitary, hypothalamus, thymus, and ovaries.

The most effective and safe range for symptoms of iodine deficiency is between 12.5 and 37.5 mg iodine/iodide based on three generations of therapeutic use by clinicians. According to iodine researchers Drs. Flechas and Abraham, women should be consuming at least 12.5 mg iodine/day, especially pregnant women who provide the sole source of thyroid hormones for their babies, which is essential for brain development and the prevention of Down's Syndrome. The Japanese consume twenty-five times more iodine than the median intake of Americans.[114]

> IODINE: A CONTROLLED SUBSTANCE—The CDC-inspired ban on iodine began October 25, 2009, and affects all 27 EU countries. The restrictions affect outdoor enthusiasts, military personnel, and travelers who, for centuries, have safely used iodine to kill parasites in drinking water, prevent thyroid disease, and prevent goiter. In the 1940s, the American diet had 800 µg of iodine. Today, the diet averages 135 µg iodine, an 83 percent decline.

IODOPHOBIA: FEAR OF IODINE

Medical iodophobia is the unwarranted fear of recommending and using inorganic, non-radioactive iodine/iodide. This fear brought about government restriction of iodine under the Recommended Daily Allowance (RDA) set at 150 µg/day. Doctors believe that more than 200 µg/day, or 0.2 mg, is toxic to the human body.

The Food and Nutritional Board at the Institute of Medicine sets a safe upper limit of 1,110 mg iodine daily, while others set an upper limit of 3,000 to 6,000 mg/day of iodine. Doctors' perceived fear of iodine traces back to a scientific experiment on rats published in 1948 called the Wolff-Chaikoff Effect, which erroneously concluded that iodine at "high" doses of 2 mg, or 20X the RDA, caused hypothyroidism and goiter. Actually, the opposite was true. The rats never became hypothyroid but instead showed improved thyroid function upon becoming iodine sufficient.[115]

> WOLFF-CHAIKOFF EFFECT—Misinformation about iodine was spread through the Wolff-Chaikoff study conducted at University of California at Berkeley in 1948 resulting in the removal of iodine from the food supply. The study, later referred to as the Wolff-Chaikoff (W-C) Effect, says that iodine intake of 2 milligrams or more is excessive and potentially harmful. The study results were never validated and have since been disproven by Dr. Guy Abraham, in his article, *The Wolff-Chaikoff Effect: Crying Wolf?*

The Wolff-Chaikoff myth was extrapolated to humans and resulted in the removal of iodine from food and water supplies. This aversion to iodine persists even today in the medical community despite numerous studies that have discredited the faulty study.[116] Ironically, even Wolff and Chaikoff admitted that iodine therapeutically treats thyroid dysfunction.[117] However, the WHO believes an iodine intake > 200 ㎍/L should be avoided in populations because they "may be at risk for developing iodine-induced hyperthyroidism."[118]

> *Of all the elements known so far to be essential for human health, iodine is the most misunderstood and the most feared. Yet, iodine is the safest of all the essential trace elements, being the only one that can be administered safely for long periods of time to large numbers of patients in daily amounts as high as 100,000 times the RDA.*
>
> — *Dr. David Brownstein*

Because most people today are loaded with toxins, iodine supplementation can cause detoxification known as the

Herxheimer reaction, which can expresses as acne, rashes, fever, headache, nausea, or diarrhea. These symptoms are due to the forced excretion of halides such as bromide, fluoride, and chloride, which are pervasive in food, water, and pharmaceutical drugs. For this reason it is important to build up iodine gradually.

> Toxic Halides—Bromine, chlorine, fluorine, and perchlorate excrete slowly from the body since there is no known liver detoxification pathway for them. But excretion can improve with high-dose iodine, high-dose vitamin C, mineral salt baths, and sweating in a dry-heat infrared sauna

Of all the trace elements, iodine is the only essential halide. Historically, it is the only halide that can be safely ingested in amounts up to 100,000 times the RDA.[119] For example, in 1911, people consumed 300-900 mg daily without incident; this is over 2000 times the RDA.[120] Patients with skin lesions, syphilis, and chronic lung infections used potassium iodide safely in amounts of up to 6000 mg/day for many years. [121] [122] [123]

Iodine safely kills malignant cells via apoptosis without harming healthy cells, while chelating metals. Taken daily in a form such as Nascent iodine at a daily dose between 6.25-50 mg, people gain a general sense of well-being, mental clarity, and increased energy. Taken therapeutically as Iodoral® in amounts of 50-150 mg iodine/day, fibrocystic breasts and polycystic ovaries reverse in women. Because low thyroid function is associated with Type 2 diabetes, 12.5 to 100 mg iodine/day can reduce the need for insulin in Type 2 diabetes. At 1000 mg/day, iodine has been historically used for life threatening infections.

IODINE IS CRITICAL FOR LIFE

- eliminates toxic halogens from the body

- modulates cardiac rhythm and blood pressure
- regulates estrogen production in ovaries
- supports immune function
- modulates pH to promote homeostasis
- reduces mucus and detoxifies lymph
- modulates blood glucose levels
- prevents cancer in breast, ovaries, uterus, prostate, ovaries, lung, and thyroid.
- prevents and reverses fibrocysts in breasts, uterus, ovaries, prostate , pancreas, thyroid
- desensitizes estrogen receptors
- prevents toxic liver and kidney conditions
- chelates mercury and other toxic metals
- protects against radiation
- destroys pathogens, molds, fungi, parasites, malaria, influenza

HISTORY OF IODINE THERAPY

Goiter dates back to Roman times when medical treatment involved either burning the thyroid with acid or cutting it out. Given current medical treatment options for Graves' disease, utilizing radioactive iodine and resection, it appears that not much has changed.

Iodine therapy had its origins under Chinese physician Ke-Hung (AD 281-361), who first used seaweed in the treatment of goiter.[124] Little was recorded in history until the late 1800s and early 1900s, when physicians prescribed elemental iodine as a supplement. In 1819, Swiss physician Jean Francois Condet first used tincture of iodine, 250 mg/day, in his practice to successfully treat goiter.[125]

In the 1820s, French physician Jean Lugol found that binding iodine to potassium made it water soluble and antiseptic. He later combined 5 percent elemental iodine with 10 percent potassium iodide in 85 percent water, at doses of 12.5 mg to 37.5 mg elemental iodine, to treat a wide variety of infectious conditions, including goiter.[126]

American pioneers who drew attention to the problem included David Marine, who in 1909 cured goiters in trout and went on to reduce the incidence of goiter in teenage girls in his "Akron Experiment" in Ohio, between 1917 and 1922, by supplementing with potassium iodide. Dr. George Goler, in 1923, used iodized water to treat an epidemic of goiters occurring in Rochester, NY, and Dr. David Cowie, in 1922, organized the first Iodized Salt Committee, which landed iodized salt on kitchen tables by 1924.

Both American and European physicians continued to prescribe Lugol's solution to treat thyroid conditions and reverse goiters before World War II, using doses higher than 2 mg daily as a preventative and cure and without adverse effects. In the early 1960s, iodine was added to bread as a dough conditioner. One slice of bread contained a full day's RDA of 150 µg of iodine,[127] more bioavailable than salt.

Today, Lugol's solution is still available in some places and still recommended at the same dose in the 1995 edition of *Remington's Science and Practice of Pharmacy*. More recent research has confirmed that 12.5 mg to 37.5 mg iodine is a beneficial range for whole-body sufficiency based on the iodine loading urine test.[128]

IODINE-LOADING TEST—This test is used to assess whole body iodine sufficiency by ingesting Lugol (Iodoral®) or 50 mg iodine/iodine in 24 hours. Healthy, iodine-sufficient subjects excrete 90% and retain 10%. Ten percent of 50 mg = 5 mg; this is the maximum amount the body can use each day for saturation of iodine receptors. Once replenished (3 months at 50 mg/day), a second test is recommended. Thereafter, the body needs half this amount, or 1-3 mg/day, as a maintenance dose. Higher amounts of 12.5 mg/day are based on French and Japanese traditions, but only demonstrate dose tolerance, and are only used for special circumstances. (See http://www.optimox.com/)

In the face of diminishing dietary iodine returns, Americans have become severely deficient in whole-body iodine. Several iodine researchers consider iodine deficiency to be a silent and growing epidemic and have called for a modest increase of the Recommended Daily Allowance (RDA) to one hundred times that of the current level of 150 micrograms.[129] [130] [131]

According to the National Health And Nutrition Examination Surveys I & III, a sharp decline in iodine soil levels in the U.S. since the 1930s, as a result of industrialized farming practices, is a main reason for a 50-percent drop in recent human iodine levels. Moderate to severe iodine deficiency quadrupled from 1 in 40 to 1 in 9 Americans. At the same time, cancers of the breast, ovaries, endometrium, and prostate increased.

In 1998, the *Journal of Clinical Enocrinology & Metabolism* further revealed "rates of iodine deficiency had dramatically increased in the United States over the past twenty years."

THE GOITER BELT IS NOT A FASHION ACCESSORY—The Goiter Belt describes the upper Midwestern States of the U.S. where the ground water and the soils have become depleted of iodine due to glacial melting. Iodine is plentiful in seawater, kelp, and brown seaweeds.

In the US, iodine tablets were added to water supplies in the goiter belt states to prevent goiters from developing. Tablets were later replaced with iodized salt both in the U.S. and around the world. In Michigan, where 40 percent of children developed goiters, iodine reversed the disease completely. No medication has since been able to replicate iodine's amazing results.

IODINE AND EDGAR CAYCE

Psychic and historian Edgar Cayce gave more than 14,000 documented readings of which approximately 8,500 were provided for individual health requests. He was called the Father of Holism for his ability to suggest non-invasive methods of returning the body to homeostasis. One of Cayce's readings, #25336, describes iodine as one of the basic elements in the body:

> Knowing the tendencies, supply in the vital energies that ye call the vitamins, or elements. For, remember, while we give many combinations, there are only four elements in your body—water, salt, soda, and iodine. These are the basic elements. They make all the rest! Each vitamin as a component part of an element is simply a combination of these other influences, given a name mostly for confusion to individuals, by those who would tell you what to do for a price.

WITH A GRAIN OF *IODIZED* SALT

When iodized salt was introduced in 1924 to reduce goiter, this form of iodine did nothing to address the rest of the body's needs or to prevent the symptoms of subclinical hypothyroidism prevalent today. That's because the body absorbs less than 10 percent of inorganic iodine found in table salt. Iodized salt is iodine mixed with sodium chloride. In its processing of salt, all trace minerals that work with iodine are removed and replaced with the additives ferrocyanide, talc (a carcinogen), and silica aluminate, designed to make salt free-flowing. Aluminum contributes to neurological disorders, especially in the absence of selenium, which is necessary for the body to chelate aluminum, mercury, and other toxins.[132]

The 1950s saw doctors reverse themselves by recommending a low-salt or no-salt diet for their "heart healthy" campaign. However, sea salt, with its grey color, contains the same mineral profile as human blood. Sea salt contains boron to prevent osteoporosis and calcification of the pineal gland, chromium to regulate blood sugar levels, and copper to help form new arteries when main arteries are clogged. In small amounts, sea salt is selectively toxic to pathogens, and lowers blood pressure. However, sea salt by itself may not be enough for people who have extreme iodine deficiencies caused by fluoride toxicity, bromism, and other known thyroid-inhibiting exposures.

IODINE REVERSES FIBROIDS AND CYSTS

Today, few physicians talk about iodine deficiency. However, according to author Donny Miller, "In the age of information, ignorance is a choice." The truth is there has been no significant clinical research on iodine therapy or use for more than 40 years. Out of sight, out of mind. [133] [134] [135] [136] [137]

What we do know? The thyroid requires only three percent of total body iodine. Of the rest, seventy percent goes to muscles and fat, twenty percent to skin; the remainder goes to the ovary and breast tissue. Each breast will grab 100-200 cc compared to the thyroid at 8.3 cc. But the thyroid gets first choice. If the thyroid is not able to meet its iodine needs, the breasts are out of luck.[138]

The ongoing epidemic of thyroid disease suggests that the body is not getting the minimal three percent of iodine it requires. Holistic doctor, David Brownstein, author of *Iodine, Why You Need It, Why You Can't Live Without It,* utilizes iodine therapy to help his thyroid patients reduce or eliminate the need for thyroid hormone. Supplementing his patients with a combination of potassium iodide and iodine, known as Lugol's solution, he observed that iodine supplementation produced the positive side effect of eliminating fibrocystic disease. While the mainstream news ignores this significant finding, it bears repeating that iodine therapy can reverse and prevent breast and ovarian fibrocysts.[139]

Dr. Brownstein and other iodine researchers noticed that roughly eighty-four percent of women with thyroid disease also have fibrocystic breasts. In practice, when thyroid patients with Fibrocystic Breast Disease (FBD) were brought to iodine sufficiency, fibrocysts in the breast and ovaries melted away. The opposite also holds true. The more severe the deficiency of iodine, the greater the number of ovarian cysts.

> In the body, human hair follicles are direct targets of thyroid hormones T3 and T4 which stimulate the production of melanin for pigment.

Cysts of Polycystic Ovary Syndrome (PCOS) are actually follicles that have undergone partial development but have not ovulated because they are starved of iodine. Iodine deficiency leads to cyst formation in the ovaries. When both iodine and thyroid function are restored, cysts reverse.

The fact that every cell has receptors for thyroid hormone means we are built for iodine. When thyroid receptors have sufficient iodine, or potassium iodide, their sensitivity to thyroid hormone is increased. As more thyroid hormone binds to the receptor, symptoms of disease disappear. Brownstein's work supports previous research showing iodine's therapeutic mechanisms of action may be at least three-pronged: hormonal, biochemical, and genetic. Dr. Brownstein explains:

> The relationship between hypothyroidism and breast cancer have been known for over one hundred years… there is a direct relationship between breast cancer and regions of the world where iodine is deficient.[140]

FBD affects 1 in 5 women and PCOS affects ten percent of women of childbearing age.[141] Both FBD and PCOS are known precursors to cancer. Thus, it makes sense to look deeper for the cause of cancer without burying our heads in the sand. Thirty years ago, when iodine consumption was twice as high as it is now (480 µg a day), one in twenty women developed breast cancer. Today, one in five women will develop breast cancer during her lifetime.

> IODINE DEFICIENCY AFFECTS ORGANS SIMILARLY—Swollen ovaries are analogous to a swollen thyroid. Both equate to hormonal imbalances:
>
> Thyroid = hypothyroidism
>
> Ovaries = infertility and PCOS.

Today, 1 in 5 men develop prostate cancer. Like breast cancer, prostate cancer has experienced the same dramatic rise in incidence and growth pattern, as well as the same response to surgery. Tumor removal does not cure cancer and can serve to spread cancer cells to other areas of the body.

A study of radioiodine uptake in two groups, women with and without FDB, revealed that the FDB breasts were able to take in 12.5 percent of the iodine dosage compared to only 6.9 percent in normal breasts. This proves iodine depletion in the breasts of women with FDB.[142]

Iodine supplementation also helps people with fibromyalgia, Peyronie's disease, attention deficit disorder (ADD), parotid duct stones. It also helps those with acute, subacute and chronic infectious conditions, immune system dysfunction and deficiency syndromes. It helps to alleviate obesity and constipation, and helps protect against nuclear fallout, industrial pollution, and reduction of oxidative stress.[143] Yet, iodine therapy continues to be ignored in favor of synthetic hormone therapy.

HORMONE THERAPY & CANCER INCREASE

The failure to properly diagnose thyroid disease as iodine deficiency has brought about an increased risk of breast cancer worldwide. This becomes obvious when comparing the rate of iodine deficiency seen in 1 of 5 women, based on urine iodine screening tests, with the rate of breast cancer seen 1 in 5 women.

Endocrinologist and iodine researcher Guy Abraham observed that synthetic thyroxine therapy in the presence of an underlying iodine deficiency increases the risk of breast cancer and thyroid cancer.[144] Similarly, a 1976 *JAMA* study concluded that "Not only was the incidence of breast cancer twice as high in the group taking synthetic thyroxine (12.1 percent in supplemented group vs. 6.2 percent in controls), but the incidence of breast cancer for women taking synthetic thyroxine for more than 15 years was much higher."[145] Other studies demonstrate an inverse relationship between iodine and breast cancer and suggest a protective role of iodine in normalizing breast tissue.[146] [147] [148]

In fact, several large studies have shown inherent dangers in hormone replacement therapy:

- The Women's Health Initiative (WHI) study, the largest study of its kind that followed women on estrogen hormone replacement therapy. This 2002 study was prematurely halted due to evidence of an increased risk of breast cancer and heart disease.[149] The investigators warned against the long-term use of hormone replacement therapy in healthy postmenopausal women.
- A 2010 follow-up WHI study further showed a statistically significant increase in breast cancer risk in postmenopausal women on combined hormone therapy (estrogen plus progestin). Women on the combined hormones were twice as likely to die of breast cancer than those women receiving a placebo.[150]
- A 1976 JAMA study found a 200 percent increased risk of breast cancer in women who took thyroid hormone

for at least 15 years as compared to women who did not take thyroid hormone.[151]

Iodine deficiency increases the risk of goiter and thyroid nodules which can lead to thyroid cancer.[152] Dr. Guy Abraham believes thyroid hormone therapy should only be considered after iodine stores have been restored. Dr. Brownstein agrees: "Thyroid supplementation increases the body's metabolic needs and therefore increases the body's need for iodine."[153]

RADIATION RISK

The elephant in the room is the sudden rise of electromagnetic frequency (EMF) exposures never fully studied for safety before being unleashed on Earth. A 2014 Israeli study showed evidence of a link between changes in thyroid cell function and exposure to nonionizing, electromagnetic radiation (NIER) related to cell phone use.[154] A similar study showed a link between cell phone use and parotid gland tumors.[155]

In Canada, the incidence of thyroid cancer is the fastest growing cancer among 15-29 year old women, as seen between 1981 and 2009.[156]

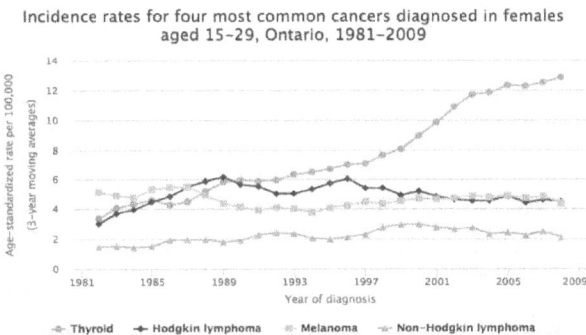

Incidence rates for four most common cancers diagnosed in females aged 15-29, Ontario, 1981-2009

Source: Cancer Care Ontario (Ontario Cancer Registry, 2012)

Figure No. 5

In the twenty years leading up to 2002, papillary thyroid cancer soared by a whopping 240 percent to become the third most common cancer in the United States.[157] According to a 2014 Korean study published in the *New England Journal of Medicine* (NEJM), thyroid cancer is the most common type of cancer diagnosed in South Korea.[158]

TRENDS OF SELECTED CANCERS IN WOMEN FROM
1999 TO 2014 IN KOREA

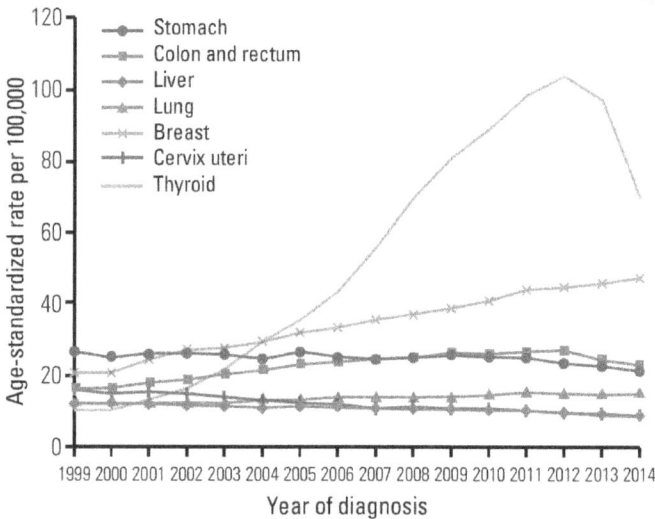

Figure No. 6 (Credit: Cancer Res Treat 9 March, 2017
| https://doi.org/10.4143/crt.2017.118)

While study authors often attribute the rise to "better screening" or "over diagnosis," the mutations noted for papillary cancer (i.e., RET gene mutations) are acquired later in life due to exposure to radiation.[159] Even with the dramatic rise in thyroid cancer incidence in less than a generation, conventional doctors still hold to a belief that disease comes through the genes. If true, how would they attempt to explain a similar increase of hypothyroidism in cats?[160] How do they claim a genetic link unless they also accept that genes adapt to our changing environment?

Thyroid disease rates are rising too fast to be based solely on genetics. While the National Institutes of Health claim that iodine deficiency is rare in industrialized nations, trends show otherwise.[161]

WORLDWIDE IODINE DEFICIENCY

Thyroid disorders of subclinical hypothyroidism and thyroid cancer in adults and children is a worldwide phenomenon where the common denominator is iodine deficiency.[162] Recent national studies in Australia, New Zealand, and thirty-two European countries, Central Asia, and the United States show high numbers of iodine deficiency. A reported 285 million school-age children worldwide are iodine deficient.[163]

Under the WHO's recommendations (250 μg/day iodine):

- In Australia, only 12% of pregnant women are considered to have good iodine status.[164] [165] [166] [167] [168]
- In New Zealand, mild iodine deficiency was documented among children, ages 5-14 years in 2002. A 2005 nationwide survey showed moderate iodine deficiency and goiter in 7 percent of pregnant women.[169]
- In most European countries and Central Aisa, goiter and hypothyroidisim during pregnancy and in infants is common.[170]
- India is reported to be "one of the biggest worldwide public health problems" for iodine deficiency disorders. Mental retardation affects as many as one in 10 children in India. A National Goiter Control Program begun in 1962 continues to distribute iodized salt and monitors children ages 8-10.[171] [172]

- The Netherlands and Japan get enough iodine through seafood and kelp, and do not suffer from the health effects of iodine deficiency. However, there is a high incidence of goiter and breast cancer in Mexico and Thailand where iodine intake is low.[173]

Even in regions considered "iodine-sufficient," iodine deficiency goes unnoticed because thyroid blood test indicators TSH and T4 may read as "normal" and so the epidemic continues.[174] [175] In pre-pregnant women, iodine deficiency leads to anovulation, infertility, and gestational hypertension. Low iodine status also causes abortions and stillbirths, as well Down's syndrome.

In the placenta, the deiodinase enzyme inactivates most of the maternal conversion of T4 to reverse T3 to ensure a significant supply of thyroid hormones to the fetus,[176] [177] which further demands an increased thyroid hormone production by the mother. Therefore, pregnant women who are hypothyroid are likely to produce children with hypothyroidism.

ADHD & IODINE DEFICIENCY

Thyroid hormones are essential during early brain development and maternal thyroid hormones are required before the onset of thyroid hormone production by the fetus.[178] [179] Therefore, abnormal levels of maternal thyroid hormone due to iodine deficiency during pregnancy may disrupt neurocognitive development in the fetus.[180] [181]

Iodine deficiency in pregnant women leads not only to IQ deficits of 10-15 points in their children, but also to hyperactivity disorder (ADHD).[182] A letter to the Editor in the *Journal Thyroid* reported that from 2001-2006, eighty percent of pregnant women and eighty percent of women of child-bearing age were not supplementing with iodine. During that same period, over

85 percent of lactating women were not taking a supplement containing iodine.[183]

In 2009, over 16 percent of public school boys took a mood-altering drug based on a diagnosis of ADHD a neurobehavioral disorder. Yet, there are no biological test markers to prove the cause of ADHD and many doctors believe it to be a 'fake disorder'. National estimates show 1 in 10 kids display behaviors such as impulsivity, inattention, and hyperactivity.[184] Based on an opinion of convenience, young girls and boys and are labeled with a disorder and treated differently by peers, teachers, and parents which can lead to social isolation. They are treated with stimulants drugs at record numbers which could lead to future drug addiction. Could the diagnosis and drug treatments of ADHD mask an underlying iodine deficiency?

CONGENITAL HYPOTHYROIDISM (CH)

Congenital Hypothyroidism affects approximately 1 in 4,000 infants due mainly to the mother's treatment for thyroid disease or an undiagnosed underlying thyroid condition while pregnant. Mental retardation or Down's Syndrome is often seen in areas where endemic goiter is higher than 30 percent and the mother is older than 40 years or has multiple children.[185] Iodine deficiency is the most frequent cause of maternal hypothyroxinaemia—low thyroxine concentration in blood—and, therefore, a potentially preventable cause of mental retardation in children.[186]

Infants with Hypothyroism

- Bones underdeveloped
- Puffy Face, swollen tongue
- Hoarse cry
- Cold extremities, mottled skin
- Low muscle tone (floppy, no strength)
- Poor feeding
- Thick, coarse hair that extends low on the forehead

- Large fontanel (soft spot)
- Prolonged jaundice
- Herniated bellybutton
- Lethargice (lack of energy, sleeps most of the time, appears tired even when awake)
- Persistent constipation, bloated or full to the touch
- LIttle to no growth

ACQUIRED HYPOTHYROIDISM

Acquired hypothyroidism is a diagnosis that manifests in older children and adolescents. It can go unnoticed for years, and is more common in girls than boys. Symptoms such as tiredness, mood swings, poor concentration, and small stature not only lead to misdiagnoses of ADHD, as stated above, but also a misdiagnosis of growth hormone deficiency.

The growth stunting rate—low height for age—for a population of children can provide a window identifying which children in that population are experiencing long-term nutritional deficiencies. In fact, nearly 43 percent (230 million) of children younger than 5 years of age in low-income countries are stunted.[187] In the US, while growth-stunting statistics are hard to find, information on growth hormone (GH) therapy as a treatment for short stature is not. Candidates for GH range from those with GH deficiency (14,336; 1 in 4000 children aged 4-15) all the way up to the 573,400 children with heights below the first percentile for age. Even pediatricians have noted that family concerns about children's' height have increased in recent years.[188]

Compare the 1 in 4000 figure of children with growth hormone deficiency to the same prevalence of children with congenital hypothyroidism and "NASA, we have a problem." Children have many of the symptoms of iodine deficiency commonly seen in adolescents and adults:

- poor concentration
- mood swings
- weight gain
- weight gain and stunted growth ("Buddha belly")
- weight loss
- lack of appetite
- bloating
- fluid retention
- poor circulation,
- constipation
- dry skin, keloidal scarring
- dry, brittle hair, split ends (human hair follicles are direct targets of T3 and T4 hormones).[189]
- dry eyes (concentrates in the lacrymal glands of the eye)[190]
- aching joints
- sensitivity to cold

CHILDHOOD THYROID CANCER – ALARMING STATISTICS

In the U.S., thyroid cancer is the most common childhood endocrine cancer, representing 1-1.5 percent of all pediatric cancers and 5-5.7 percent of cancers in the head and neck. Estimates show that 5 percent of all thyroid cancers occur in children and adolescents[191] with incidence of thyroid cancer in children up 25 percent during the past 30 years. This is significant since it seems to follow the trend for adult thyroid cancers, which is now the fastest growing cancer in the US.[192] Not surprisingly, pediatric thyroid cancer in adolescents is also associated with juvenile autoimmune thyroiditis.[193]

Although thyroid nodules in children are rare before

adolescence, thyroid nodules in children have a 26.4 percent risk of becoming cancer and childhood thyroid nodules are 4 times more likely to be diagnosed as cancer than adult nodules.[194] Thyroid carcinoma is 2-3 times more common in females.[195]

Follicular adenoma is the most common cause of solitary thyroid nodules in the pediatric population; however, solitary nodules in children reportedly have a 20-73 percent incidence of turning to cancer.[196] [197] [198] Malignant lesions are usually papillary and follicular carcinomas.[199]

Adult autoimmune conditions related to thyroid insufficiency include: anemia, cardiovascular disease, Types I and II diabetes, Addison's disease, Cushing's disease, Premature ovarian syndrome, Alopecia, Raynaud's syndrome, Sjögren's syndrome, Chronic fatigue syndrome, Psoriasis, Scleroderma, Rheumatoid arthritis, Systemic lupus erythematosus, Multiple sclerosis, and Vitiligo. However, the real health crisis shows up in our kids.

Of the developed world, American children have the highest rates of asthma, allergies, SIDS, leukemia, Diabetes Type I, and thyroid cancer, to name a few. Forty-three percent, or 14 million out of 32 million children, suffer from chronic illness or neurodevelopmental disability.[200] Nine million children have skin allergies. Eight million children have respiratory allergies.[201] Seven million children have asthma.[202] Five million children have a learning disability.[203] One in four is diabetic.[204] One in thirty-two is autistic.[205] None suffer from a deficiency of synthetic drugs.

Chapter Eight

Goitrogens

Tap Water Toxicity | Bromism | Mercury | Vaccines
Medications | Pesticides/Plastics | Isoflavins | Metals | Gluten
Intolerance | Glyphosate | Radiation (EMF) | Stress

Goitrogens are thyroid toxins with no therapeutic benefit to the body. As their name implies, goitrogens bring about goiter and thyroid disease by blocking iodine receptors. These iodine antagonists are structurally similar to T4 hormone and affect thyroid hormone responsive genes. The problem is that goitrogens are used heavily in our food and water supply and are ubiquitous in our environment.

We eat, drink, inhale, inject, implant, and absorb a chemical soup of toxins. Thyroid-inhibiting compounds are found in public water supplies, genetically-modified foods, dental materials, medications, vaccines, pesticides, diagnostic tests, soy products, breads, and hand sanitizers. They also include radiation and electromagnetic energies. Toxins defy the body's natural terrain and leave us vulnerable to disease and victims of our environment. When managing Hashimoto's or any autoimmune disease it is important to know the reasons to avoid the triggers that cause flare-ups.

ANTI-THYROID DRUGS

Many drugs affect thyroid hormones to cause hypothyroidism. The obvious anti-thyroid medications prevent the thyroid from producing excess thyroid hormones. The consequences of these drugs play out in the symptoms of fever, joint and muscle pain, nausea, swelling, numbness, headache, and liver toxicity, which can result in death.[206] Patients are prone to infections due to lack of iodide to leukocytes,[207] which reduces their rate of oxygen consumption to directly impact thyroid activity.[208] Lithium, used as a treatment for bipolar disorder, also suppresses thyroid function, as do fluoridated antibiotics.[209] Since thyroid disease can masquerade as depression, many women are prescribed anti-depressants instead of receiving a proper medical evaluation. If you are depressed, request that your medical doctor take a closer look at your thyroid, or find someone who will.

HALOGENS

Of the five halides on the periodic table of elements, iodine is the only one that is beneficial to the human body. The others—chlorine, bromine, fluorine—are toxic. For instance, chlorine in the public water supply kills bacteria but does not clean water from chemicals. Chlorine combines with chemicals to form chloramines, which are hazardous. Yet we drink chlorinated water, swim in chlorinated pools, use chlorinated detergents and plastics, and take chlorinated and fluoridated drugs. Polychlorinated biphenyls (PCBs), dioxins, and organochlorine pesticides (DDT) are all goitrogens. They persist in the environment and accumulate in fatty tissue.

Perchlorate, found in air bags, fireworks and rocket fuel displaces iodine and can damage the iodine transport system and lead to cancer. Perchlorate is so pervasive in surface water supplies due to rocket fuel contamination that it is also found in dairy and human milk. In areas with detectable levels of perchlorate, infants are found to have depressed thyroid function. Only when the body gets enough iodine are these toxins excreted.[210]

PERCHLORATE—Unsafe levels have been found in water supplies in 35 states and researchers estimate 20-40 million people are exposed.

TAP WATER TOXICITY

Possibly the largest threat to thyroid health is through forced medication of fluoride through the public water supply. Most municipal water supplies fluoridate water with a toxic waste byproduct of the phosphate fertilizer industry known as hydrofluorosilicic acid (HFSA).[211] HFSA contains significant amounts of arsenic and leaches lead from municipal infrastructures and residential plumbing. Tap water presents a 30 percent increased risk for hypothyroidism when compared to areas that do not fluoridate.[212] In the U.S., where hypothyroidism is epidemic, fluoride levels average 0.7 mg/L in the public water supply.[213]

Sodium fluoride is also used in toothpaste to "prevent tooth decay" and in infant formulas, even with a poison warning printed on the product label. Baby formula mixed with fluoridated water increases the change of developing the faint white marking of dental fluorosis. Dental fluorosis is associated with reduced IQ at fluoride concentrations as low as 0.7-1.2 mg/L, yet there is no easy way to monitor a daily dose from all exposures. [214] [215] Fluoride is a known neurotoxin in the same category as lead, mercury and arsenic[216] and listed as a Schedule 7 poison and a Corrosive 8 toxin known to damage skeletal, endocrine, and nervous systems.

Ninety percent of digested fluoride is absorbed through the intestines and distributed throughout the body to blood plasma, soft tissues, and bone where it can remain for years. In healthy individuals, fluoride is removed by the kidneys and by calcifying tissues. In people with kidney dysfunction, fluoride causes cardiotoxic effects including calcification and hardening of the arteries.[217] Since the pineal gland is a calcifying tissue like teeth and bones, it can be hardened by fluoride, which affects the onset of puberty, the sleep cycle with reduced melatonin levels, and impairs the higher functions of intuition and spiritual development, since the pineal is also known as the gateway to the Soul. Iodine supplementation displaces fluoride from thyroid receptor sites.

BROMISM

Both low and high concentrations of bromide have been implicated in thyroid disease.[218] Bromide levels can be 50 times higher in thyroid cancer than in normal thyroid tissue.[219] Symptoms of bromism include fogginess, sleep abnormalities, abdominal cramps, anxiety, anorexia, blurred vision, coma, constricted pupils, convulsions, cyanosis, diarrhea, dizziness, dream changes, hearing loss, heart beat malfunction, headache, weakness, tremors of the tongue and eyelids, muscular cramps, nausea, renal damage, kidney cancer, respiratory difficulty, salivation, slow pulse, seating, tearing, vomiting, and psychiatric, cognitive, neurological, and dermatologic disorders.

Bromine is found in breads "enriched" with potassium bromate and soft drinks such as Gatorade.[220] Unless strawberries are organic, they are sprayed with brominated pesticides. Brominated drugs are sold as sedatives, antihistamines, asthma inhalers, and even some cancer drugs. Bromine offgases from TVs, computers, copy machines, laser printers, cars, clothing, as well as mattresses and baby products made with flame-retardants in polyurethane foam.[221] It is also found in toothpaste, mouthwash, and cosmetics. Overtime, bromide accumulates in the body and bromide dominance develops.

BROMIDE DOMINANCE—Increased bromide exposures cause dangerous levels of iodine depletion. Many people are so depleted that they no longer have any tolerance for taking iodine supplements without taking appropriate precautions, such as detoxifying the body of toxic halides to open receptors to iodine. Without open receptors, iodine simply passes through the body without acting.

High bromide levels can inhibit iodine enzyme metabolism. In the 1960s iodine in bread was replaced with bromine. Breast cancer risk rose from 1 in 20 to 1 in 5.

Studies on veterans from known bromide exposures showed mild to severe symptoms of "self-neglect, fatigue, sluggishness, memory impairment, irritability or emotional instability, depression, as well as the more severe symptoms of hallucinations and violent behavior."[222] In 1946, four types of bromism were described, from simple sluggishness to delusions, hallucinations, and schizophrenic-like psychotic behavior.[223] Iodine, at high enough doses, displaces bromine from thyroid receptor sites.

MERCURY TOXICITY

Mercury toxicity is widespread throughout the world population. As an endocrine disruptor, mercury accumulates in all the glands. The body sequesters mercury in our glands where it does the least short-term damage to keep it out of the bloodstream. Mercury is especially toxic to the thyroid because it blocks selenium from binding to the enzyme that converts T4 to T3. Mercury prevents the parathyroid glands from efficient calcium, phosphorous and D-metabolism. Like fluoride, mercury reduces melatonin levels in the pineal gland to affect sleep. Mercury also damages adrenal function.

"THIMEROSAL® FREE"—Under an FDA rule change, vaccine makers can exclude Thimerosal® on the label as an ingredient if not used as a preservative, even if it is still added in the manufacturing process. Thimerosal® is ethylmercury which passes through the blood-brain barrier to accumulate in the brain as inorganic mercury.[224]

Mercury is a neurotoxin, found in dental amalgams, sodas, air emissions, makeup, in tuna fish as methyl mercury, and in multi-dose vaccines. In dental fillings, mercury continuously emits vapors. Since amalgam fillings are located in close proximity to the thyroid and parathyroid glands, they pose a major health risk. Chewing gum and drinking hot liquids can increase exposures from mercury vapor to exceed health standards by 500 percent.

In vaccines, mercury is present as Thimerosal® at 25 μg in the multi-dose flu vaccine[225] and in bundled pediatric vaccines.[226] There is little difference in the neurotoxicity of ethylmercury found in Thimerosal® and the methylmercury found in tuna fish.[227] A neurotoxin is a neurotoxin with known inflammatory, neurobehavioral and immunological effects.[228] A single Thimerosal-laden vaccine produces acute ethylmercury levels in the blood up to 20 days after injection.[229] In the blood, ethylmercury binds with hemoglobin and travels to the brain.[230] In the brain, mercury creates free radicals, inhibits critical enzymes, and impairs DNA repair ability."[231]

Ethylmercury converts to ionic mercury Hg+ which impairs the ability of the immune system to go after pathogens and parasites.[232] Mercury causes chronic, low-level brain inflammation and depression. Mercury also raises testosterone levels, which blocks a cell's ability to make glutathione to excrete mercury from the body.[233] There is no safe level of mercury exposure established. However, it is important to consume enough chelators, such as iodine, sulfur, selenium, silica, and glutathione, which bind to mercury and carry it out of the body. Ionic footbaths and infrared saunas also assist the body in carrying metals out of the body through the skin. Chelation therapy from qualified doctors can also safely remove mercury from the organs and brain for greater recovery.

VACCINES

There is no safe vaccine. However, since the mid-1960s, the CDC has been allowed to promote vaccine injection as "disease prevention." No single or bundled vaccine has been tested for safety or effectiveness beyond 72 hours prior to FDA-approval. Yet, the vaccine schedule of 79 doses by age 17 continues to expand. While the CDC claims that combining vaccines are "safe and effective," a review of the data from the Vaccine Averse Event Reporting System shows that combining childhood vaccines in one visit is not safe.[234]

Vaccines contain aborted fetal tissue cells, or human diploid cells.[235] Cell lines from aborted human fetuses have been used to develop the Rubella, Hep A, Chicken Pox, Shingles, Rabies, and Adenovirus vaccines. By injecting aborted fetal protein into the body, we prime the body to become allergic to human protein. That means vaccines make us allergic to ourselves. A 2014 study published in the *Journal of Public Health and Epidemiology* found a correlation between an upsurge in cases of autism and widespread use of vaccines made with fetal tissue cells.[236] Because fetal cell lines divide rapidly and degrade over time, they are tumorigenic. They create cancer. Knowing this, how do we consent to such procedures?

Vaccine makers genetically modify vaccines by using enteroviruses such as EVD-68 as part of the manufacturing process. According to Novartis patent EP2301572 A1, Enteroviruses and Coxackie viruses are used in both the inactivated Polio vaccine and the Oral Polio Vaccine Since 2013, these viruses have been implicated in outbreaks of paralysis similar to polio called Acute

Flaccid Myelitis. IPV is given to children four times before they enter kindergarten.

Global - Polio and Acute Flaccid Paralysis (AFP)

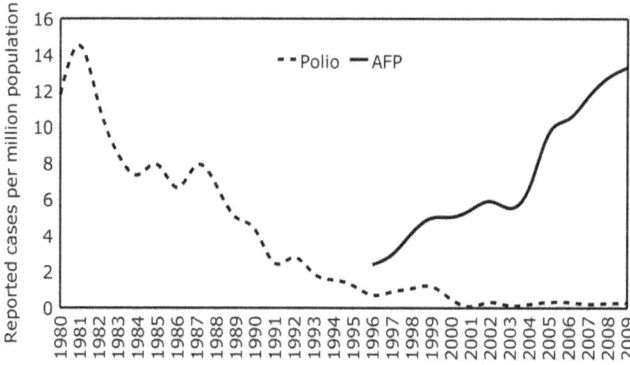

© 2011 Greg Beattie
Sources: WHO for Polio and AFP data
US Census Bureau for population data

Figure No. 7

In 2014, the outbreak of a new paralytic respiratory illness tied to enterovirus-68 spread across the Midwest,[237] coinciding with the onset of school vaccinations. A common theme emerged: Only children vaccinated with MMR, influenza, and polio appeared to be affected. Similarly, an increased risk in acquiring non-influenza-type respiratory infections was observed in those who received the inactivated influenza vaccine.[238]

Vaccines transmit highly virulent pathogens in the population through shedding, where the vaccine becomes a vector of viral transmission to cause disease.[239] [240] Vaccine package insert lists viral shedding for live vaccines such as polio, measles, mumps, rubella, rotavirus, chicken pox, shingles, and influenza, which essentially spreads the disease it claims to prevent. The transmission of lab-created viruses, from people who consent to be vaccinated to those who do not, affects the vaccinated, unvaccinated, and immune-compromised populations.[241]

The spread of disease that creates an epidemic is called a pestilence. Ironically, bovine protein detected in the MMR and influenza vaccines is known as *Pestivirus RNA*.[242] Vaccine science creates synthetic products such as Mycoplasma mycoides JCVI-sun1.0. These alphanumeric pathogens are being "designed in the computer, chemically made in the laboratory, and transplanted into a recipient cell to produce a new self-replicating cell controlled only by the synthetic genome."[243]

For what purpose are scientists re-engineering human biology? Is it to withstand the toxic soup to which we are exposed? Are we similar to GMO crops that must be modified to withstand the application of pesticides? Is the purpose to produce better soldiers? Or is it, as investigative journalist Jon Rappoport suggests, to "create weaker and more docile and more obedient and more dependent humans?" [244]

Where is the double-blind, placebo-controlled study that represents the gold standard proving that 79 vaccine doses by age 18 is beneficial for immunity, or humanity? For those who prefer a natural alternative, the science also shows Black Elderberry syrup and probiotics beat colds, flus, and strengthens immunity.[245] [246]

PLASTICS

Plasticizers are a group of chemicals, such as phthalates, styrene, and Bisphenol A, found in compact discs, food can linings, adhesives, powder paints, dental sealants, resins, polyesters, and clear plastic bottles.[247] Chemicals leach from plastic into hot or acidic beverages, which can be tracked in urine. These chemicals alter thyroid hormones when they bind to thyroid hormone receptors since they are structurally similar. So choose glass containers in favor of plastic.

ISOFLAVINS (SOY)

The isoflavins of soy protein are naturally occurring phytoestrogens that mimic estrogen to inhibit thyroid hormone production and have been linked to serious fertility problems. [248] Soy milk given to babies and children is a risk factor for the development of hypothyroidism and goiter.

Dietary estrogens at low concentrations act like DDT and estradiol to stimulate human breast cancer cells to divide. The xenoestrogens of soy are known to significantly enhance the risk for breast cancer during growth and adolescence.[249] GMO soy also contains phytic acid, which reduces mineral absorption. By fermenting soy as temph, natto, miso, and tamari, minerals become more bio-available, therefore choose non-GMO, fermented soy if a meatless diet is preferred.

GLUTEN INTOLERANCE

People with gluten intolerance and Celiac disease are ten times more likely than the general population to develop thyroid disorders. [250] [251] [252] This group also experiences behavioral disorders such as depression and hyperactivity, which reflects the gut-brain connection.[253] The damage begins in the gut where an inciting antigen is present and travels to the brain.[254] That antigen is often blamed on gluten from commercial wheat products that have been hybridized.

Most thyroid patients who follow a one-year gluten withdrawal plan feel better.[255] Thyroid antibodies disappear in the blood[256] [257] and symptoms associated with poor absorption improve.[258] [259] [260] However, even after one year on a gluten-free diet, antibodies can still be measured in the intestine, in people with ongoing inflammation. Blood tests are not sensitive enough to identify inflammation due to gluten intolerance since they only identify the end point of intestinal villi destruction as Celiac's disease. By then it's too late to prevent the damage.

Fortunately, there is a non-invasive stool test that is five to seven times more likely than a blood test to identify antibodies since the markers of inflammation; secretory IgA, along with T cells, are stationed in the intestinal mucosa. A stool test, developed by Dr. Kenneth Fine, MD, gives an early diagnosis of gluten sensitivity— before the villi are gone [261] This highly sensitive "poop test" is not offered by a medical doctor, but is available by ordering it online at Enterolab.

Embracing this idea of an environmental trigger such as gluten or radiation as a cause of internal inflammation, brings us full circle, back to the 1800s, when French biologists Bernard and Bechamp insisted that illness was a result of immune system breakdown in which nutritional status and toxicity played key roles.

The medical answer to the toxic effect of gluten is to treat the symptoms through drugs, colon resection surgeries, or the surgical replacement of bacteria via a fecal transplant. A fecal transplant transfers waste from one person to another. Why not, instead, address the root cause through a protocol that includes: 1) eliminating gluten, 2) healing the gut using healing foods such as bone broths, 3) adding herbs such as Oregon grape root, which contains berberine to close the "tight junctions" in damaged gut epithelial cells,[262] 4) using bentonite healing clays to restore the medium for gut flora, or 5) going back to unaltered wheat, the way our ancestors grew it?

Even a study from the journal *Clinical Gastroenterology and Hepatology*[263] showed that wheat made with sourdough lactobacilli, the friendly bacteria found in yogurt, rendered bread non-toxic.

A State Of Glyphosate

The real reason people are in a state where they can no longer tolerate gluten is not because wheat has been hybridized. The reason is that wheat has been poisoned with glyphosate. Glyphosate is the active ingredient in Monsanto's Ready Roundup® herbicide that is sprayed on wheat as a drying agent prior to harvest.

Glyphosate is a synthetic amino acid that mimics glycine, which is part of the cell membrane of every cell in the body. As glyphosate accumulates, it impairs cells to cause connective tissue disorders such as Lupus, chronic kidney disease, and COPD. In both animal and human tissues glyphosate causes intestinal and gut damage, specifically disrupting a metabolic pathway found in plants and bacteria. Monsanto officials will claim their herbicide targets plants, and that humans are not plants. However what they neglect to say is that humans are connected to plants at the level of our bacteria. The bacteria of plants are the same bacteria we harbor, the same bacteria that make up our mitochondria, the powerhouse of each cell.[264] [265]

Genetically modified foods contain glyphosate that act as an environmental freight train to create holes in the gut wall, killing our beneficial gut bacteria, and derailing digestion. Glyphosate makes the gut more permeable to toxins and microbes. Toxins pass through the blood-brain barrier as the brain becomes more permeable. In response, the body produces antibodies against its own myelin, the protective covering of nerve cells. This process releases opioid-like compounds capable of causing mental distress.[266] This is one reason common symptoms of thyroid disease include brain fog, loss of memory, and depression. Removing wheat/gluten not only reverses autoantibodies in thyroid disease, but also in all autoimmune diseases.[267]

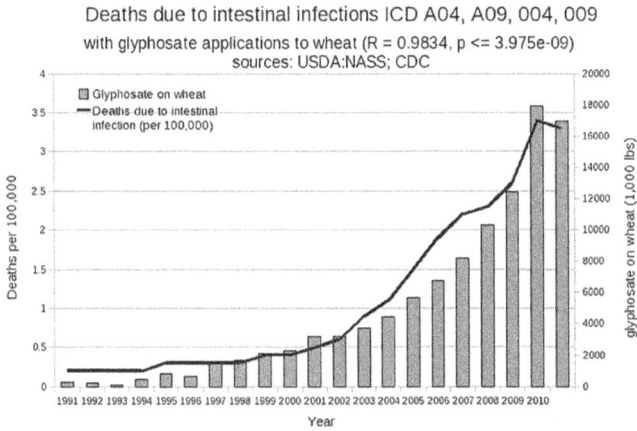

Figure No. 8 : (Credit: Samsel, Anthony & Seneff, Stephanie (2014).
Glyphosate II Samel-Seneff Toxicology FNL.)

Glyphosate is pervasive in the environment but most people don't know that it is also found in the global vaccine supply.[268] [269] Therefore, it is no surprise that it is now found in breast milk at levels up to 1600 times higher than restrictive European standards.[270]

STRESS RESPONSE

Stress is at the root of all dis-ease. When you "stress," you put yourself in a state of fight, flight, or freeze. Stress triggers the pituitary gland to increase production of its hormones, which stimulates the adrenals to release the hormones adrenaline, epinephrine, norepinephrine, cortisone and cortisol.

These hormones help to increase energy, boost blood sugar levels, and speed up circulation and respiration to help the body through fight or flight in order to survive.

However, high cortisol levels from chronic stress block glucose from getting into the tissues to cause high blood sugar. It inhibits white blood cells to suppress the immune response. Excess cortisol decreases liver function and its ability to clear excess estrogen.

It is catabolic and destroys the delicate one-celled lining of your digestive tract leading to "leaky gut" to cause poor absorption and digestion of food.

High cortisol decreases TSH, which lowers thyroid hormone production. Cortisol further blocks the conversion of thyroid hormone which can result in the body making too much T4 or the conversion of T4 into rT3.

Fluctuating levels of the thyroid hormone will throw the thyroid between a *hypo* and *hyper* state. As the thyroid swings back and forth, looking for iodine in the body, it can swell to create a goiter. Chronically high cortisol levels rob the necessary building blocks of thyroid hormones in order to better deal with the stress and eventually throws the thyroid into a permanent *hypo* state, which can lead to profound hypothyroidism.

RADIATION AND TOXIC FREQUENCIES

Rising exposure to electromagnetic radiation is a global problem. We are all part of a biological experiment without our informed consent. Future generations and the survival of Earth are at stake; we are forcing a slow migration of people out of cities to the countryside for their own survival.

Wi-fi is frying people where they sleep unless they unplug. The accumulation of hazardous frequencies from wireless utility meters, cell towers, cell phones, smart meters, and electronic appliances that now contain a 5G chip are blanketing our neighborhoods and homes with dangerous levels of full spectrum radiation. Radiation from telecommunication and 5G technologies damages our DNA, the web of our being. It is responsible for neuron damage, holes in the blood-brain barrier, and rising cancer rates.

Despite what we are know about radiation, radiation therapy in the form of radioactive isotope I-131 is the doctor's first course of treatment to kill thyroid cancer cells and shrink benign tumors, even though radiation also kills healthy cells wherever it binds, and can cause thyroid cancer. The use of radioiodide for Graves' disease has been linked with leukemia and other forms of cancer.[271]

Many electronic devices transmit additional frequencies in the 2 to 50 kilohertz range, the same range that disrupts the human nervous system. "Nerve block" is the phrase used in studies to describe the effect from technology designed to disrupt the human electromagnetic field since DNA vibrates at exactly the same frequency as telecommunication and detection devices such as cell phones, cordless telephones, pagers, microwaves, and radar equipment. Several studies have found strong links between cell phone use and DNA damage, the rise of brain and salivary gland tumors, memory loss, and reduced sperm production.[272] [273] [274]

Of course, the problem is how to address the crisis and still function successfully in our highly technological world. Is there life without a cell phone? Can humanity maintain integrity and harmony if the integrity and harmony of our cells is breaking down as we blindly push forward?

After the 1986 Chernobyl nuclear disaster, there was a dramatic rise in the number of thyroid cancers which caused up to a 100-fold increase in the incidence of pediatric thyroid carcinoma in the exposed population.[275] Radiation is used to induce cancer in lab rats.[276] In humans, cancers associated with radiation exposure are mostly papillary carcinoma, while those associated with iodine-deficient areas are more likely follicular.[277] [278] [279]

In cases of emergency radiation exposures such as Chernobyl, potassium iodide (KI) is recommended 48 hours prior or within 8 hours of exposure to reduce the uptake of Iodine-131 and the risk of radiation-induced thyroid cancer. This will only protect against internal iodine radiation poisoning, not radiation from cesium-137, Strontium-90 or the dangerous fission products of uranium-235 that attack other tissues and organs of the body.

Our exposures to toxins in all forms are on the rise without any call for caution by so-called experts. The Precautionary Principle states that when an activity raises the threat of harm to human health or the environment, precautionary measures should be taken even if some cause and effect relationships are not fully established scientifically. For too long we have swallowed the advice of experts and authorities and allowed scientific consensus to act as both judge and jury to decide for all of us. But there is a social responsibility to protect all life from harm.

Rising disease rates should make us question what needs to happen to take us in a new direction if we wish to preserve life on Earth. We have the ability to neutralize oxidative stress from harmful electrowaves and microwaves that bombard our bodies on a continuous basis. By turning back to Nature and using Earth's tools, including Bentonite clay, activated charcoal, fulvic and humic acid preparations, Ormus powder used by ancient cultures, Shungite, a mineraloid that blocks harmful waves, and Carbon 60 that can be ingested as an oil infusion, we can safely and naturally create coherent circuits in our bodies and our homes. At the same time, we can protect our mitochondria and detoxify the body to bring all life back to a state of wholeness.

CHAPTER NINE

GENETICS TO EPIGENETICS

Today, disease rates skyrocket as we function under false assumptions and old paradigms. Science clings to Genetic Determinism—The Gene Theory—in the mistaken belief that our DNA is the sole determinant for who we are. When we accept a diagnosis, we are led to believe we are defective, victims of our own DNA based on "mistakes in DNA replication" that change our cells from normal to abnormal.

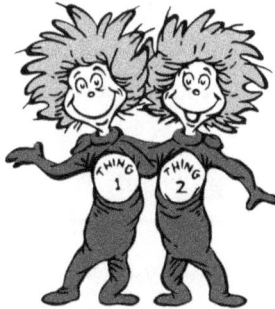

Women are increasingly victimized as *defective* through genetic branding. The BRCA1 and BRCA2 gene mutations are the new

"Thing 1 and Thing 2" of breast cancer. While scientists claim 5-10 percent of breast cancer is linked to gene mutation due to inheritance, 85 percent of breast cancers occur in women with no family history, but as a result of aging and life in general.[280] This argues that cancer is mutagenic and triggered by the environment, especially since Dr. Brownstein's work highlights the direct relationship between hypothyroidism and breast cancer, which is associated with iodine deficient regions of the world.

BREAST CANCER SCREENING RUSE

Women invited to screen using mammography should be fully informed of both the benefits and the risks. Studies are showing that screening tests for breast cancer are imprecise, unnecessary, have limited diagnostic ability, and are driving up U.S. health costs. Women who choose mammography do not know that an estimated eighty percent of breast biopsies, 1.3 million performed, result in a benign diagnosis and at a cost of $4 billion annually. Women are not told about thermography as a safe diagnostic alternative without the risks associated with radiation exposure.

A 2005 article in the *Journal Cancer Epidemiology, Biomarkers, and Prevention* found mammography increases breast cancer risk through false-positive results due to recommendations for additional tests.[281] An independent study by the Cochrane group reported that thirty percent of screenings produce false positive findings that result in an overdiagnosis and overtreatment. Overdiagnosis is a diagnosis of a condition without symptoms that would have never caused symptoms or problems. This can lead to psychological distress and anxiety. Tragically, researchers incorporate these false-positive mammogram results into models that predict breast cancer risk. [282]

Women are not only victims of false science but are also misinformed about the ionizing radiation of mammography, which contributes to mutations that lead to cancer. One mammogram is equivalent to 1,000 chest x-rays targeting one of the most sensitive tissues in the body. Further, compression of breast tissue can lead to the spread of cancer cells if they exist. This means breast cancer screenings are causing more harm than good.

Experts and agencies will not disclose that up to thirty percent of cancers naturally stop growing on their own[283] or that precancerous cervical cells revert to normal within a year and ninety percent revert within three years.[284] Few doctors know about the safe and efficient use of homeopathy against breast cancer cells.[285] Fear alone drives women to have radical surgeries to remove body parts where there is no cancer. Will women next turn to lobotomies because science has determined these same genes are also markers of Alzheimer's disease?[286]

In autoimmune thyroiditis there is a high probability of an MTHFR enzyme deficit and a Sodium-Iodide Symporter protein deficit encoded by their respective genes. However, it is important to remember that genetic changes are really epigenetic changes resulting from our exposures. For the medical world, genetic discoveries lead to drug treatments and surgeries. Meanwhile, the body is overwhelmed with metals and pathogens that need to be cleared from elimination pathways. The body requires lost nutrients to be replenished, such as iodine, boron, magnesium, selenium, copper, zinc, B-vitamins, silica, sulfur, and essential fatty acids.

The Gene Theory has long claimed that our genes predetermine our health and that disease is written in our DNA to reveal itself at some future point in time. If disease is encoded in our genes, then why does disease not reveal itself at birth? Where is the ticking time bomb gene?

Genes code for proteins using only 3 percent of DNA's full potential. What scientists are unable to explain is the remaining 97 percent of DNA—they call "junk" DNA—which is not junk at all.

Embrace your "Junk"

Few scientists pursue our "junk" because that is where genetics ends and epigenetics begins. Junk DNA is where our "switching genes" or "jumping DNA" are located to silence or activate certain genes, re-code sections of the genome, as well as modulate those switches. Our junk allows for a 528 Hz tuning fork or the sound of the voice to activate DNA and trigger healing. Our junk is where our mobile DNA interfaces with our consciousness. [287] It is where science meets spirituality.

Epigenetics goes beyond genetics to show us that our surroundings and our perceptions are more powerful and influential to health than we realize. Epigenetics explains how emotions, phobias, and traumas are passed down through our DNA right along with eye color.

When you put on your critical thinking cap, genetic theory fails to account for the fact that each of us is unique with our own ways of responding. As blueprints, genes cannot self-activate, just as a balloon cannot blow itself up. Only a signal from the environment can activate the expression of a gene. Therefore, genes do not determine whether or not you manifest disease.

Your nervous system controls the reading and modification of your genetic blueprint and carries these signals throughout the body as an extension of the brain, as well as beyond the body as an etheric sensory instrument, much like trees are sensory extensions of the Earth. In this way, the microcosm of the brain is the macrocosm of the mind where memories and experiences are found as energetic imprints in the heart and in every cell of the body. Our greatness is found in all our dimensions, from our connection to spirit to our smallest inhabitants, our microbes. If we are not aligned, then we are fighting ourselves.

Fighting Ourselves

A diseased cell is a cell without the ability to store and transport energy. Low energy transfer is caused by a unique pleomorphic bacteria which gets inside cells and blocks the production of energy in the mitochondria. Because our mitochondria represent a symbiotic relationship between an ancient microbe and human cell, what we are witnessing is a core conflict between our intracellular and extracellular microbes. In essence, we are fighting ourselves. That is our tendency in a dualistic world.

The truth is that if we create disease, we can also reverse it. The tools are presented in Einstein's equation $E = mc^2$, showing that light and matter are aspects of the same thing. We are light and shadow, the biophysical and the metaphysical, logic and creativity, intuition and rationality, ego and spirit. For full healing, we must work with all of our aspects. Only when we understand the significance of this relationship between physical and energy bodies, do we achieve multidimensional healing for ourselves.

A 2014 Italian study that kicks the gene theory to the curb once and for all showed how information passes back and forth between our cells and primary gene sequences of our genome— from somatic to germ cells—on a real time basis, and does not simply "pass down" in our genes from our parents. [288]

This study builds on earlier research performed by Russian scientists Drs. Pjotr Garajajev, Peter Gariaev, and Vladimir Poponin based on their discoveries that DNA acts like a computer chip due to its crystalline nature. At a time Americans were pouring over the Human Genome Project looking at base pairs through a microscope, the Russians focused on the vibrational nature of DNA, the ninety-seven percent scientists have termed "junk DNA," and found it to be a biological internet that not only stores information as light, but also receives, transmits, and translates it.

In their book *Vernetzte Intelligenz* translated as *Cross-linked Intelligence*, the authors explain how DNA is programmed by words and frequencies, whose code follows the same rules as human language to regenerate whole organs and to kill viruses without the application of chemical drugs.[289] They found that in living systems, chromosomes act like mini lasers to influence DNA's frequency, and the genetic information itself.

This revolutionary science means DNA reacts to language-modulated lasers, radio waves, and light frequencies if the proper frequencies are being used. Therefore, DNA is able to take up information directly from the Earth and store large amounts of information, an estimated 3 Gigabits of data, in each cell.

> *DNA is a universal software code. From bacteria to humans, the basic instructions for life are written with the same language.*
> — *San Francisco Chronicle, September 2000*[290]

Mainstream scientists have covered up the truth about our DNA. They claim, "the science is settled"—an oxymoron. Real science is never settled. Real science continues to ask questions. When we begin to connect the dots, it is no longer necessary to decode, splice, manipulate, or replace genes. We are each a reflection of our DNA and our DNA reflects us. Our DNA is really a spiral galaxy of divine light that holds memories and experiences originating from our ancestors. We carry the information of the ages within.

In the search for truth, we must reexamine the possibilities. However, learning new truths often comes at a cost. My awakening showed me that most of what is considered science today came from what was accused of being magic centuries ago. When we are open, we see that magic is merely the unseen side of life. If we can accept magic as part of *imagination*, as clearly as it is written into the word, we are much closer to appreciating our innate ability to heal ourselves. For me, a diagnosis of profound hypothyroidism led me to question my reality. As I opened to new information, I had to learn to let go of memories of who I thought I was. In the process of accepting myself on multiple levels, I came to accept that I carry the energetic patterns of my ancestors with me that manifest in the physical.

TRANSGENERATIONAL INHERITANCE

If you wonder why you share similar traumas as your parents or grandparents, it is because emotional traumas are passed down in the genome from our ancestors and translated into the body as illness. Inherited family trauma is real and manifest in the physical. In the presence of anger, hate, jealously, rage, or stress, DNA is compressed and therefore, cannot fully function. In the presence of positive emotions, DNA relaxes and is able to express.

The transfer of memories and experiences from our ancestors is called *transgenerational inheritance.* During a traumatic event, part of the soul essence can be fragmented and split off as a way to adapt and cope. The dissociated soul parts depart, carrying the pain and shock of the trauma that would be unbearable to the sufferer. Tribal societies know this 'soul loss' is meant to be temporary, but problems arise when soul loss is ongoing.

When the soul separates from the body it is an instinctive response. Symptoms of profound soul loss manifest as feelings of being fragmented, "not being all there," blocked memory, listlessness, inability to make decisions, inability to feel love or receive love from another, or can be expressed as despair, addiction, depression, or suicidal tendencies.

Emotional traumas are passed down through our chromosomes and stored in our cells. Because we are connected to our ancestors through a spiritual umbilical cord, we can be triggered generations later by a similar stressful event, causing us to reenact aspects of the original trauma in our daily lives.

Transgenerational trauma is the notion of unhealed issues of prior generations being expressed in current generations. In some cases these unhealed issues can continue for thousand of years.

— Eshowsky, Shamanic healer and author

Emotional trauma migrates to the psoas muscle (pronounced so-as), the deepest muscle in the body. According to some spiritual philosophies, the psoas is the muscle of the soul. The psoas connects spine, legs, and diaphragm to the reptilian brain, the ancient part of the brain stem. It stabilizes the spine and forms a shelf for the vital organs of the abdominal core. This bridge between emotional and physical bodies shortens under chronic stress to exhaust the adrenals and deplete the immune system.

A constricted psoas leads to pain in the low back or knees; it can cause sciatica, disc problems, hip degeneration, menstrual pain, infertility, and digestive problems. A relaxed psoas is the mark of creativity and play. It grounds the body to the Earth and rekindles energy flow by reconnecting the body to universal energy.

Psychologist Carl Jung believed that what remains unconscious does not dissolve, but resurfaces. As history shows, we tend to keep repeating our unconscious patterns until we bring them into the light of awareness. Once aware of a solution, we can stop looking at the past. When we heal energetic patterns that do not serve us, we heal them for generations going backwards and forwards through time. When we cut the spiritual umbilical cord, we heal the trauma for all time.

SOUL HEALING

Soul healing is a process not only for eliminating symptoms but also for achieving higher states of health. Shamans who do soul retrievals, work with spiritual guides in the next dimension to track soul parts and return them to the individual.

As my physical symptoms began to reverse, I was drawn to join a group of healers led by shaman Myron Eshowsky. He reminded us that, as spirit embodied, we are here to connect divine intelligence to Mother Earth for our mutual healing. Where there is soul loss, there is also soul retrieval, if the soul allows. The soul is in charge. When the emotional body suffers, the consequences manifest physically, as a wake-up call from the soul. In answer to a question on soul separation, Myron suggested:

> Soul is our core essence and it is larger than us. It connects us to the collective soul of all life. It protects against any threat to our core being, as part of an innate instinct for survival.[291]

Shamans are healers. They use creativity and art to heal themselves and facilitate healing in others. In his book, *Peace with Cancer*, Myron writes:

> An aspect of shamanic healing traditions is to either put something back that has been lost or remove an illness which has been taken on... The uniqueness of the person influences the specifics of the path taken.[292]

Shamans see healing as an art. They see or feel energy as light and move it. They free up the body's healing energy to flow. When this happens, spirit reconnects with Source and energy is freed. There is a breakthrough. From their book *Shaman Wisdom, Shaman Healing*, authors Michael Samuels and Mary Lane write, "The process of making art is the process of seeing into visionary space, the same process shaman use to see as they heal."[293]

The shaman creates a sacred space where the constructs of ordinary life are left behind to prepare to meet the divine. In this healing sphere of safety, everyone is protected. Here, the shaman helps open the heart. Heavy energies of pain and grief can be released and transformed into light so joy can be experienced. As the client tells his story, the shaman reflects it back as power and beauty so the client can "see the light" as himself. Healing is about being seen and loved. When the healing work is finished, sacred space is closed to prevent contamination.

> *The artist invents new space, where there wasn't space before, and then he creates new energies there. Artists produce unprecedented dimensions and worlds.*
> — *Jon Rappoport, The Magician Awakes*

Nature shows us how all life on Earth is interdependent for our mutual survival and our collective evolution. Our microbes, cells, tissues, organ systems, and our bodies are ecosystems that are part of a greater ecosystem working in cooperation for balance. Each level is inclusive of all the levels beneath it while also transcending them, as the whole transcends the sum of its parts. The same self-transcending principle holds true for our lives through our auric layers of the energy body. As we move outward from our physical layer to the mental, emotional, and spiritual auric layers, we resolve dilemmas at each level by going one step higher.

The body shows us that we are no more victims of our genes than we are victims of the choices we make. Our genes show us the consequences of our choices. They also show us how we change our biology. Going beyond genetics to epigenetics means that we can transcend disease and claim our rightful place as healers.

Chapter Ten

Food as Medicine

Eczema, mood swings, muscle aches, exhaustion, attention deficit, weight gain, weight loss, growth problems, digestive problems and frequent colds are the signs and symptoms of mineral imbalance. Imbalance is the picture of thyroid disease. If disease is the process of coming out of balance, then healing is the process of reintegration.

Farmers have long understood the connection between plant health and the soil. As minerals in the soil decrease, disease rates increase. Acidic soils result from the overuse of pesticides and fertilizers. If soil is too acidic, minerals dissolve too quickly and are carried away in water runoff. On the other hand, if the soil is too alkaline, not enough minerals dissolve and become bound up or "constipated." As you might guess, soil is healthiest when pH is balanced at a neutral pH between 6 and 7. The same scenario plays out in our bodies.

MINERALS GO DOWN, DISEASE GOES UP
Changes in the rates of selected reported chronic diseases, 1980–1994
(per 100,000 members of the U.S. population)

Disease	1980	1994	Percent increase	Mineral deficiencies associated with disease
Heart conditions	75.40	89.47	18.67	Chromium, Copper, Magnesium, Potassium, Selenium
Chronic bronchitis	36.10	56.30	55.98	Copper, Iodine, Iron, Magnesium, Selenium, Zinc
Asthma	31.20	58.48	87.44	Magnesium
Tinnitus	22.60	28.24	24.98	Calcium, Magnesium, Zinc
Bone deformities	84.90	124.70	46.96	Calcium, Copper, Fluoride, Magnesium

Source: USDC, 1996, Werbach, 1993

Figure No. 9

When Amish farmer, John Kemf, added important trace minerals back into deficient soil, he showed that the plants were able to defend themselves and pesticides could be avoided. He was 18 years old when he said:

The immune response in plants is dependent on well-balanced nutrition in much the same way as our own immune system. Modern agriculture uses fertilizer specifically to increase yields with little awareness of the nutritional needs of other organic functions.

We are connected to the Earth in a dynamic relationship through our microbes and our minerals. Depleted soil leads to depleted foods, which leads to depleted bodies. Foods can either harm or they can heal. They can be toxic or they can be medicinal. Often, replacing deficient foods with healing foods is the only medicine needed.

According to Chinese, Indigenous, and Ayurvedic traditions there is no clear distinction between food and medicine. However, in the west, the gulf between food and medicine has expanded along with waistlines. The majority of food is of low frequency and empty calories because the life has literally been processed out of it through commercial farming practices, pesticides, irradiation, pasteurization, genetic mutilation, chemical additives, preservatives, and added sugar. Obesity is the bloated, modern picture of starvation that illustrates our disconnection from Earth. As a result, Americans are projected to live shorter lives than previous generations lived.

The media generates a false narrative that Americans are healthier today and live longer than ever before even as disease rates rise and life spans fall. The contradictions that exist are wake-up calls to question the prevailing wisdom of food, nutrition, and medicine. The popular aphorism *garbage in, garbage out* not only describes our food, lifestyle, and behavior, but also our beliefs about who we are. In our rush to be efficient, we've traded the garden for the shopping cart, wild foods for fast foods, and agriculture for agribusiness, and in the process(ing), have lost our connection to Mother Nature.

During the mid-Victorian era, people lived significantly longer, in good health and worked until the last days of their lives without current medical diagnostics, drugs and surgeries. Granted, they had to survive the first five years, but if they did, they averaged 75 years as men and 73 years as women. The mid-Victorians benefited from eating a nutrient-rich diet which has been lost to us due to our sedentary lifestyle and food choices.[294]

Food, health, and disease are frequencies on a spectrum. When Hippocrates said, "Let food be your medicine," he was really saying, "Natural forces within us are the true healers of disease." He was talking about frequencies. Organisms use minerals of a specific frequency to support biological processes. At the wrong frequency, minerals are not absorbed. Therefore, we need to appreciate the energetics of foods if we are to grasp the key to lasting health. For a list of low and high frequency foods, see Appendix IV.

Chinese herbalism describes the relationship of healing foods to flavors that enter the different organs: Sourness enters the liver; bitterness enters the heart; sweetness enters the spleen; spiciness enters the lungs, and saltiness, the kidneys. Without all five classical flavors, imbalance can occur. No one needs to be committed to the corporate food pyramid or to any pyramid scheme, for that matter. Healing happens when nutrition is improved and toxicity removed.[295]

REMOVE, REPLACE, REINOCULATE, REPAIR

To understand food as medicine we can utilize the functional medicine model of the 4 R's: Remove, Replace, Reinoculate, and Repair.

Remove: all processed, irradiated, genetically-altered, preservative and hormone-laden foods. These foods have the life processed out of them. In addition, they include inflammatory foods such as gluten, pasteurized dairy, corn, soy, and sugar, vegetable oils, colas, caffeinated drinks, alcohol, fluoridated and chlorinated tap water, and hydrogrenated and transfats.

Replace: the nutrients, minerals and enzymes gone missing. These foods include seaweeds, ginger, pineapple, ghee, coconut oil, raw butter from grass-fed cows, avocado, cherries, beets, hemp seeds, chia seeds, flax seeds, and herbs and spices. **Iodine-rich foods** include dried kelp and sea vegetables, cod fish, navy beans, pastured eggs, potatoes, green beans, raw milk, raw yogurt, kefir, dried prunes, tuna, pastured turkey, strawberries, cranberries.

Reinoculate: with non-inflammatory, probiotic foods. Probioitic foods are higher in beneficial bacteria than probiotic capsules since they come with their own terrain. They include fermented and pickled foods, such as sauerkraut, kimchi, kombucha tea, kefir, beet kvas, and pickled beets. Non-inflammatory foods include those high in glutathione. Homocysteine is the best diagnostic measurement of inflammation. When there is high homocysteine, use **folate-rich foods** of beans and lentils, raw spinach, asparagus, romaine lettuce, broccoli, avocado, oranges, and mangoes. In cases where homocysteine is measured as low (below 6 umol/l), use the **sulfur-rich food** of whey protein. A combination of magnesium and B6 can be utilized as well.

Repair: with foods that cleanse and heal at the same time. These include foods high in minerals such as bone broths, raw honey, and apple cider vinegar. The following list represents some options for a natural "repair kit."

Natural Detox Repair Kit
Digestive-Parasites
Colon hydrotherapy

Clays of Bentonie, Montmorillonite, Illite

Activated charcoal

Slippery Elm, ginger, Cascara sagrada bark

Algin from seaweed

Fulvic acid-humic acid -zeolite

Apple pectin

Flaxseed

Silver

Ozone

Liver
Coffee enemas

Burdock root and dandelion root teas

Whey protein for glutathione

Tinctures of yellow dock, red root, ginger root

Oregon grape root, milk thistle, nettles;

Spices of cinnamon, turmeric

Warm lemon water before breakfast

Apple Cider Vinegar with the mother

Whole-food Selenium

Green juicing

Castor oil packs

Skin and Lymph

Ionic footbaths

Infrared sauna

Epsom salt and clay baths

Rebounding, skin brushing

Green juicing

Red clover tea

Lymphatic drainage

Radiation

Ormus

Carbon 60

Hydrogen-rich water

Nascent iodine, detoxified iodine, kelp

Apple pectin cilantro, parsley, chlorella, Spirulina

zeolite

Dental

Oil Pulling

For a more complete listing of culinary and medicinal foods, herbal tinctures and teas, see Appendix II.

THE SKINNY ON FATS

When healing the thyroid, it is also important to ensure a steady supply of good fats, known as saturated fats. The belief that foods must be "low fat" or "no fat" is one fallacy that needs to melt away for physical healing to happen. According to Gary Taubes, author of *Good Calories, Bad Calories*, at least fifty to seventy-five percent of your total calories should come from healthy fats.[296]

Healthy fat foods include olives, avocados, coconut oil, cod liver oil, evening primrose oil, organic pastured raw butter, cacao butter, raw nuts such as macadamia and pecans, seeds such as black sesame, cumin, pumpkin and hemp seeds, organic pastured eggs, grass-fed meats, nutrient-rich grass-fed raw dairy, lard, and tallow.

Saturated fats have been demonized even though they make up sixty percent of your brain. These beneficial fats supply sixty percent of your heart's energy. They protect your skin from the sun and make up the membrane of every cell in your body. They serve as precursors necessary to synthesize vitamin D, a steroid hormone that strengthens the immune system. Researcher Ancel Keys launched the Seven Countries Study in 1958, the first prospective study on diet, lifestyle, risk factors and cardiovascular disease carried out in sixteen populations of seven countries. Keyes tested the linear thinking of conventional medicine that cholesterol from animal foods negatively impacts human cholesterol. He found no link at all between dietary cholesterol and blood cholesterol levels. After one thousand subsequent studies later confirming his results, the case should have been closed.[297]

Yet Americans still swallow the dogma of the "cholesterol myth." The truth is, there is no such thing as good or bad cholesterol. Cholesterol is cholesterol. Cholesterol is the body's fire fighter, coming to the rescue when there is injury in the body. It is there to heal, not to take the blame for starting the fire. When the damage is repaired and the threat neutralized, cholesterol is shuttled back to the liver in HDL.

The lipoproteins HDL and LDL are the "fire trucks" that carry cholesterol and fat throughout the body. While LDL delivers cholesterol to repair the damage, HDL carries it back to the liver. Cholesterol is the precursor of important steroid molecules such as the bile salts, and steroid hormones, including vitamin D. The five major classes of steroid hormones include: progestagens, glucocorticoids, mineralocorticoids, androgens, and estrogens.[298]

Fat is not the problem. The body makes four times more cholesterol than food could ever provide. Therefore, there is no need to avoid red meat, liver, fatty fish, pastured eggs, raw, grass-fed dairy and dark chocolate as long as each is produced humanely and without chemicals, hormones, or GMOs. Saturated fat does not clog the arteries.

Saturated fats are necessary for liver function, healthy lungs, proper nerve signaling, healthy bones, slowed digestion, bile acids, and hormone production. These fats are also necessary to cushion and protect internal organs, to transport fat-soluble vitamins, and to stimulate natural immunity. You cannot live without cholesterol. You would have no cells, no skeleton, no muscles, no hormones, no bile salts to digest fat, no digestion, no brain function, no memory, no nerve endings, no movement, and no reproductive system. Furthermore, fat makes water. For every one pound of fat, the body synthesizes 1.1 liter of water. Camels, rattlesnakes, and scorpions survive desert conditions by producing water from their own fat pads.

While the FDA and the food industry continue their attack on saturated fats, eating saturated fats reverses atherosclerosis in post-menopausal women.[299] In fact, high total cholesterol levels later in life reduce the risk of dementia[300] and are predictive of a long life. In other words, people with a higher total cholesterol level live longer.[301] The bacon and egg breakfast, slathered with raw butter and cream from grass-fed cows and eaten by our grandparents, was life-giving.

The true value of saturated fat and cholesterol puts statin drugs in a new light. Statins artificially lower cholesterol to stimulate heart attacks and atherosclerosis, the very things for which they claim to prevent. [302] Statins inhibit the synthesis of K2, which protects arteries from calcification, and they lower Coenzyme Q10, an antioxidant that protects against hardening of the arteries. CoQ10 is vital for energy production in cells, especially muscle cells. Because statins reduce cholesterol, which is required for vitamin D synthesis, people who take them are also at risk for vitamin D deficiency. If sourced from food, vitamin D is best obtained from unfermented cod liver oil and raw milk from grass-fed cows. As Weston A. Price discovered in his study of traditional diets around the world, the healthiest cultures obtained sixty percent of their calories from fat. Both vitamins A and D are really fat-soluble hormones. As hormones they are self-regulating. In other words, the body knows what to do with them when they come in their natural form. Note: Avoid synthetic forms of vitamin A and D due to likelihood of toxicity. In supplementing with unfermented cod liver oil, fat-soluble vitamins A and D are balanced, so neither is toxic. Vitamin A is essential to the integrity of the epithelial lining of the gut, to maintain a healthy balance of gut bacteria in the microbiome. Vitamin D plays many roles in the immune system. Another vitamin D-rich food comes from the unprocessed milk of grass-fed cows.

GOT RAW MILK?

I stopped drinking pasteurized milk in my twenties when I suddenly became violently ill. Running to the bathroom to throw up every morning after my breakfast wasn't worth the trouble of keeping milk in my diet. Like many others, I discovered I could no longer assimilate milk because I no longer produced the lactase enzyme to digest it. The milk industry calls me "lactose intolerant" but what I later came to understand is that I was not lactose intolerant, but rather pasteurization intolerant. My body, in its wisdom, was telling me to put down the adulterated product and step away from the counter. At the same time, I picked up a book by Ron Schmidt, *The Untold Story of Raw Milk*, which explained that raw milk from grass-fed cows contained everything I needed to digest and assimilate milk because it was a whole food that has existed for centuries and has nourished civilizations. I began drinking it. I raised my kids on raw milk and watched their eczema, asthma, and ear infections disappear. We stopped seeing the doctor and I never looked back.

Raw milk from grass-fed cows contains bioavailable vitamin D to strengthen bones and the immune system. It also contains a full compliment of B vitamins, vitamin C, minerals, proteins, essential fatty acids, antibodies manufactured in the udder, and live bacterial cultures that aid in digestion. Since it contains sixty known enzymes, including lactase to break down sugar, and lipase to break down fat, raw milk has the ability to completely digest itself. People lose weight when drinking raw milk. You could call raw milk a form of border security because it contains special combat forces that provide multiple redundant systems that can reduce or eliminate populations of pathogenic bacteria and bring the microbiome into homeostasis.

Medical thought in the 1900s embraced holism, as doctors prescribed raw milk as medicine. William Osler, MD, considered to be the world's most influential figure in the history of medicine,[303] used raw milk from pasture-fed cows, rich in butterfat, to treat the chronic diseases of the nervous system, heart and kidneys; he used it to treat high blood pressure and edema, as well as rheumatic fever and stomach cancer. In almost every case, he recommended high quantities of raw milk. Patients were told to rest in bed and were given milk in small quantities totaling five to ten quarts a day at half hour intervals. Hot baths, hot packs, and a daily enema were also given.

In 1929, Dr. J. R. Crewe, a physician at the Mayo Foundation, published "The Milk Cure" in *Certified Milk Magazine*. Crewe wrote, "When sick people are limited to a diet containing an excess of vitamins and all the elements necessary to growth and maintenance, which are available in milk, they recover rapidly without the use of drugs and without bringing to bear all the complicated weapons of modern medicine." [304] Raw milk is called white blood because it not only resembles blood but also makes blood. Blood is the catalyst of metabolism.

The message from the FDA today is this: "Raw milk is inherently dangerous and should not be consumed." [305] However, raw milk is direct competition against a declining dairy industry monopoly. The pasteurization process destroys all enzymes, beneficial bacteria cultures, vitamins, minerals, and essential fatty acids, while adding unregulated fillers to milk. Processed milk is dead milk since it must be sterilized to compensate for acidosis the cows develop from a corn-fed, junk food diet. Deficiencies in cows are translated into deficiencies in the humans who drink processed milk and then express symptoms such as allergies, intolerances, and digestive disorders. When pasteurization does not work, illness and death can result. The largest multistate bacterial outbreak in 1985, which sickened over 200,000 people and killed 18, was traced to pasteurized milk. [306] Many other outbreaks of pasteurized milk are also reported. [307 308 309 310 311]

When it comes to the body's vitamin D needs, only ten percent comes from food. That's because our bodies create the most bioavailable vitamin D3 in the skin through the action of the sun's UVB rays on cholesterol. And that requires high enough cholesterol levels from our diets.

As Nature intends, the sun is the best source of vitamin D3. During the summer months, and depending on the latitude, it is possible for a full ninety percent of our requirement to come from the sun. This is confirmed by studies showing people who sunbathe safely, for limited periods, without sunscreen live longer and have a lower risk for cardiovascular disease than those who do not.[312] People with light skin should take care to limit sun exposure to twenty minutes during midday, or until their skin begins to turn pink. If we can achieve our nutritional needs through a combination of whole foods and the sun, why then are more people today supplementing with vitamin D as a synthetic isolate? For more information on the association between D-deficiency and thyroid disease, and why synthetic vitamin D supplementation is not a good idea, see Appendix III.

VEGETABLES AND JUICING

Some vegetables, when eaten in large quantities, are thought to interfere with iodine metabolism. These include soybeans as well as the Brassica vegetables such as broccoli, cauliflower, kale, rutabagas, radishes, turnips, cabbage, and Brussels sprouts. Because all vegetables are healthy, it is always recommended to rotate them in meals to ensure that you receive all the phytonutrients the body needs. Since plant phytochemicals protect plants from disease, injury, and pollution, it is no coincidence that people whose diets are high in phytonutrients have a low incidence of disease.

In autoimmune disease, digestion is impaired due to leaky gut. One way to bypass the digestive system until the epithelium "tight junctions" can heal ... using bone broths and other foods ... is through juicing. Juicing allows liquid nutrients to go directly to cells where they can produce energy. If the digestive system is functioning poorly, then so are eliminatory organs. Juicing is highly detoxifying because it supports liver and kidney efficiency.

One way to improve kidney function is to drink celery juice. Celery's organic mineral salts and enzymes naturally nourish blood, increase hydrochloric acid in the stomach for improved digestion, and help to resolve ammonia permeability. Juicing celery also helps support adrenals, neuron functioning, and thought patterns. Celery's electrolytes hydrate cells and repair DNA. If that is not enough, celery is one of nature's greatest healing foods for bones as it contains high levels of calcium and silicon.

HEALING CLAY REBUILDS MEDIUM FOR FLORA

Autoimmune thyroiditis benefits from healing clays, which may be human's earliest example of using Earth's resources as a natural medicine. Native cultures from Africa to North and South America all recognized the healing benefits of clay, whether applying it topically, bathing in it, or ingesting it in small amounts.

All healing clays are a crystal matrix and have the ability to act as transducers once they are properly hydrated. Their nanoparticle size, their shape, and their electromagnetic properties make clays an important tool in any healing toolkit. Today, clay is commonly used to reduce food and mercury poisoning, promote digestive health, provide trace minerals, support immune and lymphatic systems, and eliminate internal parasites. It is used to repair and heal. In his book on clay for healing purposes, Raymond Dextreit writes:

> Excess gas often happens due to a deficiency of the right intestinal flora to process fat, flour products, and cellulose during the last phase of digestion. Problems can persist until enough good flora can be reconstituted. Clay helps rebuild the medium for the reconstitution of flora and prevents growth of pathogenic bacilli. Clay coats and tonifies an irradiated gastric wall, stimulates the liver, balances stomach acid, and purifies the colon.[313]

Clay holds a negative charge that binds to positively charged toxins and pathogens to carry them out of the body. Clay can be safely ingested in small amounts as a medicine because it is colloidal, homeostatic, and living earth.

As we evolve forward to reclaim the idea that food is medicine, we will be going back to the garden, back to the kitchen, and back to basics. At that point, the FDA will become obsolete. For a list of traditional foods and herbs to build the immune system and help reverse thyroid disease, see the Back to Basics list I compiled in Appendix II.

CHAPTER ELEVEN

BE YOUR OWN HEALER

All are us… the dualistic dream starves the spirit and gives rise to the gamut of illness of the body and soul. The job of medicine, then, is to nourish the spirit by bringing people into the source of wellbeing—the dream of nature.
—Eliot Cowan, Plant Spirit Medicine

A healing evolution is available to us if we choose it. We are our own healer because healing is an inside job. The capacity to heal comes not from a book, an institution, a law, or a doctor with a degree. We are healers simply by virtue of having been born. Choice is vital to the process of healing because the power to heal comes from the freedom to choose.

CHANGE THE WORLD YOU OCCUPY
Our choices don't change the world, but change the world we occupy. Since our world is malleable and not solid, there are many probable worlds, each based on how we perceive it. Perception changes as we change since we see only what our current view holds; whether it is the duality or nonduality, the reductionist

medical view or the holistic natural view, the victim or the innovator.

A nondualistic view shows us that each of us is a spark of God, a fractal of the whole, a mini universe in relationship with the greater Multiverse. When we open to the nature of the divine, we open to healing.

In Nature, there is no duality, no separation, no destruction, and no force. Nature is a cycle of change during which steady states, such as death, are only temporary. From cells to seasons to solar systems, everything is in flux, expanding and contracting, rising and falling. The evolutionary cycle of existence—birth, adaptation, death, rebirth— shows us who we are. We are non-linear, with no beginning and no end. Each of us can name little deaths we've experienced as we leave old patterns behind to embrace new ones. My own experiences show me that the greatest transformation comes when I hit bottom. Crisis creates opportunity.

In *Shaman, Healer, Sage*, Alberto Villoldo writes:

When we get sick we have the opportunity not only to regain our health but to make a quantum leap to an even greater level of wellness. Healing is a method of not only eliminating symptoms but for achieving increasingly higher states of health.[314]

Everything in Nature is interconnected for our mutual benefit. We see how a plant communicates its medicinal relationship to the human body through its form, color, shape, function, and terrain under the "law of similars." For instance, the stinging nettle is known to cause pain from its defensive stinging hairs if you brush against its stems. Most people would call it a weed and ignore it. The Native Americans, however, have used nettle for centuries as a counterirritant against pain by striking the affected areas of the body with its branches. They use nettle root decoction for painful stiff joints, and they rub powdered nettle leaves on limbs with rheumatism.[315]

Nature is abundant with remedies. Plants, trees, streams, lakes, animals, birds, reptiles, and humans are all spirit expressing themselves through individual forms for mutual healing. Plants are plant-spirit medicine, water is water-spirit medicine, humans are human-spirit medicine, and so on. Nature is made up of the elements, each with its own spirit medicine.

THE ELEMENTAL ARCHETYPES

Each element, down to its atomic level, has a material and a spiritual aspect. On a physical level, elements can be toxic, neutral, or beneficial. On a spiritual level they are all gifts.

The work of Barbara Brandt, founder of the Atomic Messages Foundation, builds on the science of the 118 elements and adds a deeper dimension. Brandt describes the elements of the Periodic Table as personalities that express both an imbalance and a gift. Each personality is a vibration that heals its own imbalance. As with homeopathy, whose foundation is "like cures like," each element-remedy is able to transform a person's negative symptoms into that element's positive state.[316] This gives meaning to the phrase, "the answer lies within." Each element shows us how we are our own healers.

Atomic archetypes show how the elements work on a quantum level. Based on intuitive readings, Brandt's work offers a roadmap of unique personality patterns for the 118 elements in the Periodic Table that reflect a specific spiritual quality. The seven rows correspond to the seven chakras. Row one, containing hydrogen and helium, is related to the qualities of the first (root) chakra. Row two, containing lithium, beryllium, boron, carbon, is related to the qualities of the second (sexual, relationship and creativity) chakra, and so on.[317]

PERIODIC TABLE OF THE ELEMENTS

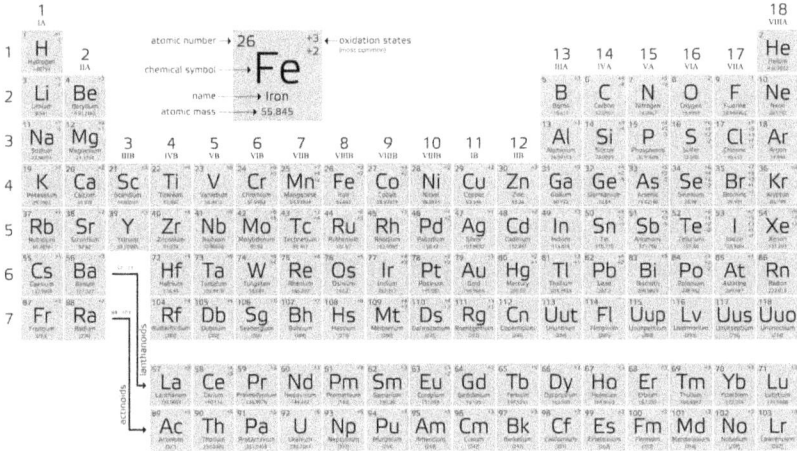

Figure No. 10

Similarly, the eighteen columns of the Periodic Table represent a wave of rising and falling activity. The elements in column one represent "New Beginnings." They rise to a peak of activity in column 10, and then gradually fall back down to rest in column 18, which represents "Turning Inward and Resting."

Personality Patterns of the elements in Columns 1 and 2 are related to Water, symbolizing new possibilities and new beginnings; Columns 3, 4, 5, and 6 are related to Wood, symbolizing active growth; Columns 7, 8, 9, and 10 are related to Fire, symbolizing a peak of energetic activity; Columns 11, 12, and 13 are related to Earth, symbolizing harvesting; Columns 14, 15 and 16 are related to Air/Metal, symbolizing letting go; and Columns 17 and 18 return to Water, symbolizing resting. The Noble Gases of row 18 don't mix with other elements; they rest.

Years after I healed my thyroid, I sought out a homeopathic doctor to help resolve an energetic block. To my surprise, he devised a constitutional remedy from the Periodic Table of the Elements. Listening to my story, the homeopath identified a pattern of giving up my power to authority that could be traced back through my mother to Nazi Germany.

My homeodynamic remedy contained the imprint for several elements: Pt, Fe, Fr, Cs, K, Rb, and Na including milk remedies from the horse and the cat. People who take milk remedies have a tendency to crave comfort foods, which could come from a lack of infant feeding or poor bonding with the mother. They may be fussy about eating or missing a meal, as if they are "empty" both physically and emotionally. They may be self-conscious or shy. People who take lac felinum are cat enthusiasts. What they love about cats is their independence. On the other hand, lac equinum, or horse milk, reflects a feeling of being overwhelmed by duty and the hardship of life, as well as an intolerance for injustice.

A major theme in Lac Equinum (mares milk) is a feeling of having one's wild spirit or nature beaten out - of being tamed into submission. This was expressed in the proving as the frustration resulting from a large, wild animal having been subjugated, domesticated, selectively bred, and, too often, mistreated by humans. Think for a moment of the battles in which horses were sacrificed, of rodeos and racetracks, slaughter houses, and overburdened pack horses.
— *Nancy Herrick, Animal Mind, Human Voices*

Vibrational medicine has the benefit of giving a deeper insight into soul essence. I didn't question the remedy. Because the subtle effects of energy medicines are experienced on many levels, they are impossible to measure in a linear way. Each individual is a composite of experiences that are impossible to separate.

I took two doses of the remedy twelve hours apart. Within four weeks, I began to notice a subtle difference in how other people responded to me. Six months later, I followed up with a second remedy containing Krypton, whose message is to unleash the voice within by listening to inner guidance to know what is right.

Homeopathy may have originated before 400 BC, pre-Hippocrates. A homeopathic remedy is made by a homeopathic pharmacy using repeated dilutions of a specific substance extracted in alcohol or water called a "mother tincture." After each dilution, the mixture is strongly shaken to create increasing potencies until little or no substance remains. The dosage forms: X(1:10 ratio), C(1:100 ratio), M(1000C), are pellets composed of sugar and lactose saturated with the liquid dilution and labeled with the dilution-based potency. This 'minimal dose' medicine acts as a stimulus to the body's vital force to bring about healing on multiple levels. Substances can be plants, bugs, minerals, just about anything in nature. Those with thyroid disease will, no doubt, appreciate knowing about the gift of iodine and its archetype.

THE IODINE ARCHETYPE

Iodine sits in the 5th row of the Periodic Table, corresponding to the 5th chakra, for expression, and in the 17th column, corresponding to understanding reality as a paradox, seeing the big picture, connection, compassion, health, and separation.

In her book, *The Atomic Messages of Peace, Love, and Healing*, Brandt describes the Iodine *Archetype* as one of compassion, laughter, humanitarianism, and empowerment for victims who suffer. An imbalance in iodine creates victimhood, a sense of "Why did this happen to me? How did people in power let this happen?"

Iodine's *Message* is to understand the whole process—the building up and breaking down—and to be willing to let it go. Be willing to look at the bigger picture before acting. For self-protection, it is important to use humor, laughter, and detachment to prevent yourself from becoming a victim.

Iodine's *Gift* reminds us that people who suffer have their own potential power to heal, so it is important to avoid seeing them as victims. It is important to help those who suffer to empower themselves while maintaining our own power and clarity.

Give a man a fish and you feed him for one day; teach a man to fish and you feed him for a lifetime.

— *Proverb*

Since the 1940s, scientists have created forty-three new elements. Regardless of the origin, whether natural or artificial, the elements are connected to their own spiritual energy patterns, messages, and unique spiritual gifts if we are open to receive them. They can assist humanity with the gifts of appreciation, compassion, empowerment, and deeper insights.

This compassionate side of the elements is naturally downloaded into all of us. We express their gifts, which come and go depending on the circumstances of life. Brandt writes:

It's not a coincidence that Hydrogen, the first element in the Periodic Table, represents "the Ongoing Creator of New Ideas"—new ideas that can then be materialized.[318]

New ideas are needed if we are to reverse epidemics of blood sugar imbalances, hormonal imbalances, food intolerances, chronic stress, and digestive disorders that describe the epidemic of thyroid disease.

Thyroid disease is an imbalance due to a breach at every level of existence. The loss of integrity in the cell membrane leaves us open to physical attack in the same way a breach in the aura leaves us open to psychic attack, in the same way a nation's open borders are vulnerable to foreign attack, in the same way a breach of contract leaves an individual open to exploitation. The world mirrors what's happening inside. At the core of all imbalances is fear.

FEAR OF CHANGE

Change is the only constant in an evolutionary process. However, the fear of change is endemic in a world of duality where separation, conflict, and isolation thrive. Perhaps it is not change per se that people fear, but rather the process of stepping into their healer shoes. After all, it is easier to trust the experts than to trust themselves; easier to fear an invisible virus than to trust in the power of the immune system; easier to be co-dependent than interdependent, easier to be the victim than the innovator.

> *The huge population of viruses, combined with their rapid rates of replication and mutation, makes them the world's leading source of genetic innovation: they constantly "invent" new genes. And unique genes of viral origin may travel, finding their way into other organisms and contributing to evolutionary change.*
>
> *— Villarreal LP. Are Viruses Alive? Scientific American, December 2004.*

Viruses are innovators. They use the tools available to them to ensure the survival of their species. Fear is not an option. If we allow ourselves to be innovators, without fear, then humanity, like the virus, ensures its own survival. Self-healing requires us to transcend fear to embody love, to transition from a material world to the heart. In our material world, fear manifests as the lower frequencies of anger, aggression, domination, disharmony, scarcity, victimhood, unworthiness, and dependency. In the heart, love manifests as the higher frequencies of joy, self-love, caring, harmony, abundance, self-worth, and freedom. Each of us gets to choose.

HEALING THE VICTIM

To heal a victim mentality, we must stop playing small. In a world built from systems designed to isolate human beings through conflict, artificial intelligence and digital technology, the heart remains the final frontier, untouchable, and our most powerful tool for change. The heart radiates an infinite power of love that cannot be derailed because it is a direct line to our divinity.

Creating a heart-based culture requires us to write, speak, dance, sing, and act from the heart. It requires us to be sensitive to our emotions. The driving force of the heart is caring. The world we occupy will change only when we care enough. Change comes from giving a damn and from being compassionate to others. It also comes from loving ourselves enough to maintain healthy boundaries. We must accept ourselves unconditionally, flaws and all, to shift the victim complex.

When I stopped resisting, I allowed the healing to happen. When I stopped attacking myself emotionally, I stopped creating antibodies against myself. Reconnecting with Nature freed my body to heal itself. To know Nature is to know freedom; you cannot have one without the other. As my body cleared, so did my mind. I saw what passes for authority as the illusion of an unsustainable system. Any ecosystem that grants itself authority over the divine will of others is an ecosystem outside Nature and Natural Law.

The choices we make come from divine will, which comes from the soul. The soul is the driving force for growth at the level of the cell. In gaining body consciousness, the soul loses consciousness to be slowly reawakened in the physical. When we awaken to see that body and soul are one, it becomes important to treat your body as a temple of the soul. To nurture the body-soul is to eat clean foods, drink clean water, clear out toxins, and be clear about your intentions. When you love your body and work with it, it miraculously works with you. This is the model relationship for working with others. Working through the heart is how miracles are created. The heart is where love finds a home.

For me, the effect of freeing my body to heal itself changed my view. On one level, I was no longer a vibrational match with my partner, who worked as a medical doctor. On another level, I reignited my desire to go in the direction of my passion, which led me to enroll in a degree program at Trinity College of Natural Health in Naturopathic Medicine.

Sometimes our lives have to be completely shaken up, changed
and rearranged to relocate us to the place we're meant to be.
— *Author Unknown*

VOICING TRUTH

As caretakers and overachievers in home and the workplace, women tend to give up energy to others at their own expense. They hide behind their own shadows. The systems of education, religion, politics, medicine, government, and media all tell women it is their job to be selfless. Women believe it and create it. Women have been conditioned to feel guilty if they put themselves first, so they choose to be last. It is a belief system that usurps all other systems and creates a victim class of females.

Our beliefs stem from our views about ourselves, which create the world we occupy. By suppressing our gifts, we occupy our own private hell on Earth. It is our resistance to our nature that takes us out of alignment with health, wealth, joy, abundance, power, and freedom. We pinch ourselves off from the flow. Only when we stop hating ourselves, stop fighting ourselves, stop dividing ourselves, do we learn the lessons that end the pain so we can occupy heaven on Earth.

Voicing my truth was my medicine. In order to break through to the next level, I was provided opportunities every step along my way. Divine guidance led me to friends who supported me and offered me a platform where I could share my truth on live radio, in podcast interviews, and in front of an audience. I knew that if I had said no to the offers, the well would have run dry. So I let go of any preconceived ideas and learned to trust the process. I asked for assistance when necessary and let my passion propel me in the direction of my calling. I decided to ride the wave of experience without defining it. Each opportunity provided a chance to receive and to give back. Healing is about relationship, and realizing that opportunity is on the other side of fear.

Sometimes the best things happen when we least expect it. Healing happens when we can become vulnerable to the experience. When we open the door of the heart and walk in to merge with the light of our inner truth, we free our voice. Centered in our truth—we are no longer held captive to a story we create about ourselves. When there are no more excuses, it is time to wake up to the wisdom of the heart to identify with higher states of health. We become the architects of the life we wish to build. We only need to reclaim responsibility and choose to play the part.

Chapter Twelve

The Power OF Relationship

What we see happening in our environment reflects what is happening inside. Our relationships with our children, partners, colleagues, clients, politicians, doctors, religious leaders, educators, communities, governments, and nations all mirror the relationship each of us cultivates within ourselves. The individual reflects the whole.

A nation out of balance reflects an imbalance within. A parasitic culture, in which politicians lie, steal, and cheat show us the culture of our own constitution. Parasites require a host to survive since they cannot live independently. They take without giving back. They stimulate adaption of the host environment to come into balance or both will die. For parasites to be present we have chosen to give up our power to settle for less.

A loss of power can manifest in individuals as manic-depression, medically diagnosed as "bi-polar disorder." Bi-polar is someone with a dissociative disorder who lacks a strong sense of self, unable to withstand the tension of opposites. If we asked our microbes how to heal from such resistance, to make peace with the perceived paradox, they would tell us to understand the conditions that caused the disconnection in the first place.

Examples of Contrasting Qualities

- Accepting vs. Rejecting
- Admitting vs. Denying
- Aware vs. Preoccupied
- Cheerful vs. Manic
- Concerned vs. Judgmental
- Confronting vs. Harassing
- Conscious vs. Unaware
- Giving vs. Taking
- Healing vs. Irritating

- Holistic vs. Analytic
- Honest vs. Legal
- Impartial vs. Righteous
- Intuitive vs. Literal
- Spontaneous vs. Impulsive
- Surrendering vs. Worrying
- Tender vs. Hard
- Trusting vs. Gullible
- Virtuous vs. Celebrated

The contrasts of duality work in our favor if we can use them as tools to make better choices. The ability to make good choices happens when we take time to slow down, to get quiet, and let the soul remember its mission. This happens when we are centered in our personal power, without being isolated in it. Being centered means we are connected to something larger, a microbiome within a biome within an ecosystem.

A healthy and balanced dynamic that we share with our microbes is the same we share in all our relationships. If we can "deconstruct the diagnosis" for our bodies, we can reconstruct a new world for all. But we must be willing to drop the victim label and see ourselves as innovators. As innovators, we hold the blueprint for our lives. We are responsible for our actions. Our lives have no meaning unless we meet our needs directly, which always involves taking responsibility and taking action.

Fortunately, life is full of thorny dilemmas that allow us to practice being innovators through the prism of relationships. If we can step back and see the greater story, then each thorn can serve to sharpen our perception to see the options for healing. Whether we choose to see our thorns as a setback or opportunity determines whether we hobble or waltz along our path.

THE THORNS OF SELF-SACRIFICE

Problems are only opportunities with thorns on them.
         — Hugh Miller, Scottish writer

In a world of contrasts, too often we are convinced that self-sacrifice is the ultimate contribution to the whole. We buy into the paradigm of giving at our own expense. Each sacrifice becomes a thorn. When we hold tightly to these thorns, we not only limit our potential for growth, but everyone else's, too. Stagnation becomes the norm and history repeats itself. A thorn in the paw impedes progress.

For instance, when people give up eating meat for the cause of "animal rights" and suffer physical ailments as a result, neither they nor the animals benefit. For the cause to be virtuous, the relationship must benefit all bodies—the person, the animal, and the Earth. Therefore, a better choice than abstaining from meat would be to restrict the amount, and eat only from animals raised locally, naturally, and humanely.

The dilemma to end my marriage provided no risk-benefit calculation, no map, and no book on the subject to guide me. I took a leap of faith to self-discovery and let go. I released resistance. I began living in 'the now' while letting Source take care of 'the how.' As I tugged on my thorns, questions arose: *How would I meet expenses? How would my kids handle the transition? Was I being selfish?* In surrendering to the experience, I trusted the journey of the soul. I saw myself as the switch giving power to a future of my making.

Our questions take us to the heart and soul of our dilemmas.

If we give up value to others without real returns, we deplete our reserves. If we give up our wellbeing, we end up losing ourselves. Without clear emotional boundaries, we lose our inner resolve along with our health, a lose-lose proposition.

He tended to deny his own needs in order to fill the needs of other people. An imbalance with the love of self and others. He felt so passionate about his work and messages, subconsciously speaking, that he was putting himself on the back burner. That's what caused all the heart issues that Mr. Carlin ultimately faced.

—*Lisa Caza, psychic on comedian*
George Carlin, Outer Limits Radio

In every case of self-sacrifice, we choose suffering as a badge of honor only to cripple ourselves. By holding onto the thorns out of a perceived obligation, life becomes a burden, too overwhelming to bear. We become the crutch that holds others up at our own expense. Habitual patterns are self-inflicted thorns that prevent us from healing. At no time do we affect change in another person or in society as a whole unless we are willing to change our view, from self-sacrifice to self-love.

If the foundation is cracked, you don't paint over it, you build a new foundation. If you bypass the affliction, you not only enable a self-limiting pattern in others, you drive your own thorns deeper, as well. For me, the complete shutdown of my thyroid provided an opportunity to change my perception. It propelled me to leave the foundation of a home I helped construct in order to come home to myself.

In her book *When Things Fall Apart: Heart Advice for Difficult Times*, Pema Chödrön writes:

Nothing ever goes away until it has taught us what we need

to know. If we run a hundred miles an hour to the other end of the continent in order to get away from the obstacle, we find the very same problem waiting for us when we arrive. It just keeps returning with new names, forms, manifestations until we learn whatever it has to teach us about where we are separating ourselves from reality, how we are pulling back instead of opening up, closing down instead of allowing ourselves to experience fully whatever we encounter, without hesitating or retreating into ourselves.

The patterns we continue to experience are spiritual, karmic lessons in the greater story of our mutual healing. I call karma 'the Law of What Goes Around Comes Around.' What you put out, you get back in *this* life—a continuous energy exchange in real time. Life does not happen in the past or in the future because the past is past, and the future never arrives. Life happens in the now, in real time, just as our own cells transfer information from somatic to germ cells—on a real time basis. The lesson of karma is about being responsible for your choices and accepting the consequences of those choices. The lesson is about showing up.

If we can reset the dynamic with the relationship with the self, we also reset the dynamic in our relationships with others, which ripples out to our communities, governments, other nations, and the Earth. Such a profound shift cracks a whip through space and time as the world we occupy reorders itself. As the dust settles, we move forward together in a new resonance and harmony.

We are all in this life together, playing different roles on a continuum for the evolution of the soul and of the whole. The whole is only as strong as its weakest link. Thus, the greatest betrayal in life is ignoring the self. If we can change our perception to see that our divinity connects us to all life, then our thorns fall away. When we free our thorns, we free ourselves for the healing that wants to happen.

In order to bring balance and freedom to our lives or to a nation, we must see ourselves as our microbes do, as part of a symbiotic whole. The body frees itself from disease by targeting infected cells while creating new ones: self-editing and self-regenerating. Listening to the body's innate wisdom means we heal a nation one body at any time.

Parasites show us what is happening not only within our bodies but also within our minds. Parasites reflect the falsehoods we have allowed to invade our mind and feed off our sensibilities. Under the Germ Theory of Disease, we believe the body is victim to the germ and we fail to see that our true nature that is always changing with our surroundings.

Nature shows that we heal relationships when we heal ourselves, first. We heal as individuals when we can let go of people and things that no longer serve us in favor of those that do.

> *The modern view alienates us from our innate connectedness. It is a conditioned view, not a natural one. This is good news, because the nature of a person will always be their nature, and whatever is conditioned can be unconditioned.*
> — *Eliot Cowan, Plant Spirit Medicine*

Our nature is Nature. Everything outside is a reflection of what we perceive about ourselves. Every choice, thought, and action ripples from cell consciousness to influence all life. That means that every step we take to support our light serves to support all life. What we put out we get back.

TRUST YOUR GUT

Author and shaman Robert Moss refers to dreams as the doorway between worlds. He writes in his poem, "Hunting Power," from his book *Here, Everything is Dreaming*, "You think you are hunting your power but your power is hunting you." Moss suggests that when we are unable to see our way in the waking world, our dream images put us in touch with a vast source of creativity that gives us courage to trust ourselves to heal ourselves.

Dreams give the body a story in images and scenes, depicting a drama that reflects our lives on the big screen. When we know we are living a story on a multidimensional stage, it becomes easier to cope with the daily dramas. We see how we are being guided with the tools needed to manifest the solutions in the waking world. What we fail to pick up consciously, the subconscious uploads to us. The best way to hold onto dream guidance is to write a dream down immediately upon awakening. Keeping a dream journal, over many months, will help to connect the dots of the greater story.

On my healing road, I came to a crossroads where my world drama split into five different directions: divorce, kids, health, career, and writing. When these became too much to contemplate, I turned the controls over to the Divine.

On my writing path, after years of writing young adult fiction, I failed to find an interested editor and publishing house for my book *Earth Keepers*; I filed it away and began writing nonfiction. When I submitted my healing story to the "Be The Light" essay contest, I was awarded a t-shirt as a top prizewinner. With this sign of affirmation, I decided I would write the truth of what I knew from my own experience and publish it myself.

After my husband and I filed for divorce, I chose to enroll in a holistic degree program that allowed me to stay home with my kids. Within two years, I graduated with a doctorate in naturopathic medicine and made my thesis the core of my first book, *The Nature of Healing, Heal the Body, Heal the Planet*. In opening my healing practice, I began to move my innovation forward through others.

In the process of ending my marriage, I changed the view that I had to carry the overwhelming load of making my marriage work at all costs. In putting my needs equal to others, I not only ensured that I would be there for my children, but also that I would be an example in case they should ever find themselves in similar circumstances. By trusting my gut and taking profound measures, I healed myself of profound hypothyroidism in less than a year.

> *The fifth chakra gives us the ability to envision possible futures and to act on our vision. You imagine who you can become and feel the freedom of infinite possibilities.*
> — *Alberto Villoldo, Shaman, Healer Sage*

As I saw my symptoms reverse and my thyroid hormones reach optimal levels I knew I had taken the necessary steps. Along the way, I learned to check-in with my feelings and ask myself, "Am I am stepping on thorns? Giving my power away? Activating my boundaries appropriately?" The more I trust my guidance—intuition, synchronicities, and dreams—the stronger my alignment between body, mind, soul, and spirit.

Healing happens when we become aware of the dualistic habitual patterns that hold us captive. Only when we believe we are already whole and complete, connected to everything, do we cultivate the relationship with self and revert back to a state of harmony, in balance with our microbes and the Earth.

CHAPTER THIRTEEN

EARTH KEEPERS

The living Earth and its species depend on each other for mutual survival. If we do not accept our responsibility as caretakers of our bodies and keepers of the Earth, we destroy ourselves in the process. Everything we are is also what the Earth is. If the Earth is healthy, so are we. If we are sick, so is the Earth.

For humanity to evolve under conditions of rising disease rates, growing division, and ongoing conflicts, we must honor our relationship with Mother Earth, recognizing that what we do to Earth, we do to ourselves. If we are both the biophysical and the metaphysical, the elements of the Earth and consciousness in an Earth suit, then perhaps humanity can come together as Earth Keepers.

During the Renaissance, philosophers promoted a mechanistic view of the body to justify a top-down ideology and social order as the natural order for all. [319] The human mind bought into the programming and we dissociated from Nature. We failed to appreciate our relationship with Nature, which passes messages to us through sound frequencies.

THE FREQUENCY OF NATURE, 528HZ

All of Nature vibrates at the tone of 528Hz, as one of nine creative core frequencies on the Solfeggio musical scale. Hidden within each frequency on the tonal scale is a correspondence to a color as well as a chakra.

The 528Hz frequency is the precise center of the electromagnetic color spectrum. It relates to middle C, the note MI on the scale, which derives from the phrase *MIra gestorum* from a Gregorian chant, meaning *miracle*. 528Hz corresponds to the color green, the center of a rainbow. Green is the frequency of the heart charka. It is the color of grass, trees, and phytoplankton, whose foundation is chlorophyll. Therefore, chlorophyll is a sound manifestation of frequency vibrations that takes on the pigment of greenish yellow.

The chlorophyll molecule receives the 528Hz frequency from the sun, which resonates at 528Hz. Chlorophyll is selected by all of Nature to be the principle energy carrying and transforming pigment to generate life-sustaining oxygen. 528 Hz is also the frequency known to repair DNA.

We are not separate from Nature; we are interdependent, where no species is higher than another. We embody Nature's physical elements of earth, fire, air, ether, and water, as well as the atomic elements of carbon, hydrogen, oxygen, and nitrogen. The elements show us who we are in the natural order. What if the universal healing frequency of 528 Hz was paired with the universal solvent—water—to advance the future of medicine?

BE LIKE WATER

Thyroid disease reflects a pattern of giving without being able to receive. Of the five elements, water has the feminine quality of nurturing and receptivity, since it will receive all things. "Be like water" was the advice from one of the most influential martial artists of all times, Bruce Lee:

Empty your mind. Be formless, shapeless, like water. You put water into a cup it becomes the cup. You put water into a bottle it becomes the bottle. You put it in a teapot it becomes the teapot. Water can flow or it can crash. Be water my friend.

We live in an ocean of frequencies in which water is a source of life. While we are told that the body is comprised of 80 percent water by weight, we are not told that on a molecular level we are 99.9 percent water. We are not bodies containing water; we are bodies of water in the form of human beings.

Water reflects the nature of all life because water shares sacred geometry with the universe. A water cluster is an arrangement of two or more water molecules. While two water molecules don't have much shape, as more come together they adopt various structures. Water at five molecules in its free state forms a pentagon. At six molecules, water forms a hexagonal organized matrix and is considered structured. As water interacts with higher frequencies, the geometries become more complex.

What we cannot see on the molecular level, is visually demonstrated by cymatics, the science of sound. Cymatics shows how sound and vibration move particles to create form, as seen on a metal plate. The higher the frequencies the more complex the geometries created. Cymatics provides a visual of how water is structured and matter is created out of the field of energy.

Cymatics represents a looking glass into a hidden world to unveil the substance of things not seen.[320]
— *Evan Grant, researcher*

Like our DNA, the structure of free-flowing water holds, receives, transmits and translates information as light. As we are light beings, we are also structured water beings.

STRUCTURED WATER

In Nature, water is naturally structured through the hydrological cycle and charged by the far-infrared frequencies of the sun. Photosynthesis means photon fusion or light injection. Thus, the water in raw, organic fruits and vegetables is structured so that the minerals of the soil have been transformed from inorganic to organic to hold light and become bioavailable to the body. The same is true of the healing power of colostrum brought through the mother to provide life-giving nutrients for the child. The body is designed to "add light" to the water so that food becomes medicine. This way, there is no need to drink gallons of water each day to hydrate. The body naturally transforms water into a healing elixir through the power of the sun in the fruits of the Earth. There is a difference between inorganic calcium in the soil, which is not assimilated by the body, and organic calcium of raw vegetables, fruits, and mother's milk, which is.

Water is uniquely adapted to our biology so that our cells can utilize the nutrients from food with greater ease than they can with other liquids.[321] Water's strong tetrahedral hydrogen bond network makes a flexible framework for many chemical processes to take place. Water transports materials throughout the body, hydrates cells, generates proteins and enzymes, conducts electrical signals with minerals at lightening speeds, contracts muscles, divides cells, and detoxifies by carrying waste out of the body.

When water is in the form of tap water, bottled water, mineral water, or spring water, it is unstructured and may leave people dehydrated because the size of the water molecules have not been structured. Minerals in the water are not absorbed. Unstructured water acts as a solvent. Its job is to clean out the garbage. Distilled water in its "free state" is negatively charged and picks up anything positively charged—minerals, toxins, and pathogens—and pulls them out of the body. Free flowing water is distilled because it is "not still" at a molecular level. There is no opposing charge so there is nothing to slow it down, which makes it a powerful tool in detoxifying the body. It is why distilled water is recommended for the coffee enema as a tool for liver detoxification. However, when water is structured, it is rebalanced, as it is in Nature. It brings energy back to the body because it holds more energy.

WATER MACHINES

Due to contamination of the public water supply, people are investing in various water systems for taste and purity. Reverse osmosis (RO), alkaline water machines, and molecular hydrogen water machines are three types of water systems with big differences. An RO system can remove fluoride and impurities, but its negative charge pulls essential minerals out of the body just as it pulls them out of the pipes through which it flows. If the body fails to get enough minerals, it fails to function optimally.

Most water machines that alkalinize water by shifting pH are problematic. Alkaline water only neutralizes acidic pH at the point of contact—stomach and small intestine. Drinking too much alkaline water artificially disrupts the body's normal pH. Further, minerals in alkaline water can begin to accumulate to unhealthy levels if kidney function is poor. Alternatively, there are ionizing machines that "structure" water without alkalinizing it to produce molecular hydrogen or "hydrogen rich" water to help neutralize free radicals, detoxify the body, and provide a form of water that is more easily absorbed for better cell hydration.

SYNERGY OF WATER

Though we may not realize it, we harness the power of water within us because water surrounds DNA's structure in a "hydration shell" attached by hydrogen bonds.[322] This is important since just as water influences our DNA, our emotions influence the structure of water. Our DNA changes shape based on an emotional stimulus. Whereas negative emotions such as anger, hate, rage, or jealousy compress DNA, positive emotions such as gratitude, appreciation, compassion, or love relax DNA.[323] A study by the Institute of HeartMath showed that donor and isolated DNA separated by miles have the same emotional responses at the same exact time when using heart-based intention. This shows the cells of the body are responsive to the heart's magnetic field.[324]

Another name for structured water is "liquid crystalline water" because it has communication properties similar to quartz. It carries information and holds memory, which means it holds information as frequencies in the quantum state[325] and is able to communicate instantaneously with its surroundings. The idea of "body memory" tells us that memory exists throughout the body in the form of water and pure energy.

Through his compelling water photos, Dr. Masaru Emoto demonstrates how words, intention, prayer, and emotion, transforms the atomic structure of frozen water crystals. He tested the theory that the memory of water is a fractal of consciousness with the power to restructure itself.[326] In 2008, Dr. Emoto conducted a ceremonial blessing of Lake Baikal in Russia, the world's deepest fresh water lake. Using an electrophotonic camera, sensors measured changes in electrical charges at various stages of the ceremony. [327]

Learning about water is like an exploration to discover how the cosmos works, and the crystals revealed through water are like the portal into another dimension.

— Dr. Marasu Emoto, author

All our aspects—physical, emotional, energetic, conscious— reflects the flow of water as it moves through the body, cycles through the rivers, transforms through the atmosphere, and falls back to Earth. When Dr. Emoto expressed water's relation to the cosmos, he understood that liquid crystals are phases of matter as they transition between the solid and liquid states."[328] [329] In essence, humans are embodied, polyphasic liquid crystals. Our liquid crystalline structure organizes our biology and its function as well as patterns of our development.[330]

Water shape-shifts in four phases: solid, liquid, gas, and a fourth quantum phase, or "exclusion zone," in which water holds a negative charge. Water's fourth phase allows for tunneling,[331] which happens when a particle or molecule overcomes a barrier and can be on both sides at once, or anywhere in between. In the case of water, when put under extreme pressure in small spaces, it is both particle and wave at the same time. What gives rise to this fourth phase?

According to Greg Pollack, author of *The Fourth Phase of Water*, when water is exposed to the sun, its fourth phase builds and the charges separate, suggesting that sunlight is the catalyst that drives the buildup of this phase.[332] The knowledge that water is charged by the sun for transformation has been utilized for centuries to create flower essences. The sun is critical for vitality and health of all life on Earth. Deprived of the sun, we wither and fade, or we freeze. Water's negative fourth phase is the reason for the Earth's net negative charge with its free electrons that represent a foundational element in healing the body. Grounding to the Earth, as well as ingesting and bathing in healing clays, are primordial tools that reconnect us to the Earth and awaken our healing potential.

HYPOTHALAMUS: GATEWAY TO THE UNIVERSE

The hypothalamus is the gateway gland that interfaces with the soul through four higher chakras beyond the body. Water influences the function of the hypothalamus, which in turn regulates body temperature and the flow of water.

When medical science ignores the metaphysical nature of humanity, it ignores our connection to our divinity.[333] A toxic metal body burden draws in the parasites that also reflect a parasitic culture. If we continue to consent to such an assault, we seal our fate as host and victim to industries that profit and feed off of our energy at our expense.

> *But if they're so successful, why haven't parasites taken over the world? The answer is simple: they have. We just haven't noticed. That's because successful parasites don't kill us; they become part of us, making us perform all the work to keep them alive and help them reproduce.*
>
> — *Daniel Suarez, author of Daemon*

If we are to survive, we must be the voice that speaks against injustice and in favor of the Earth and her diverse species.

> *The sky chakras are supported by the earth chakras, just as the branches of a tree are supported by its roots. The gifts of the higher chakras (6, 7, 8) are immensely practical and manifest in this world. They are not otherworldly. When Christ taught "The Kingdom of God is at hand," he implied that Heaven and Earth are one, indivisible.*
>
> — *Alberto Villoldo*

Parasites do not manifest in a body unless the conditions of the body allow them to be present. When parasites arrive they are there to clean up the mess. In order for our parasites to revert back to their former selves, we must work with them.

Sound Healing

For me, profound hypothyroidism did not manifest overnight. The suppression of my thyroid took years to evolve based not only on my exposures, but on my emotional diet as well. Only when I began to express myself did I begin to heal. In looking back, my fear went deeper than a fear of speaking. My fear came from a lack of self-worth. No one was stifling me or telling me I was hopeless, except me. No one gave up my power but me. No one but me filled myself up with empty calories—with things, people, pets— thinking they offered me a sense of security and belonging. Once I accepted responsibility for my deficiencies, I had to introspect, understand my fears, forgive myself, and move forward.

At this time in our history, humanity faces a dilemma. While we do not consent to the breach that threatens all life we can use this as an opportunity to free the voice to speak for the Earth, while using the tools of Nature. If sound can reset the rhythm of the body, then food, herbs, homeopathics, plants, and words are frequency medicines that can entrain the body back to the rhythm of Nature. All life is rhythm. Our bodies naturally take on frequencies that are missing to become harmonious and coherent. When it comes to healing frequencies, what is true of food is also true of sound.

Holistic medicine offers many options in sound healing for the human energy field, using tuning forks, gongs, crystal singing bowls, chanting and mantras, and toning with the human voice. Music therapy, alone, is often the best prescription to lift the spirit, with benefits seen in those who suffer with Alzheimer's, autism, and Post Traumatic Stress Disorder.[334] As crystal water beings, we only need to remember that when we create music with our voices, we heal, and the song of laughter is the best medicine.

We have the ability to transform and benefit all life on Earth, since all life connects through universal vital force. However, we need to balance problems with solutions. When we speak solely of 'doom and gloom,' we remain in a state of victimhood. Instead, we can live by the Precautionary Principle, a strategy by which preventive actions are undertaken before harm occurs.

We are here to express our gifts and experience life without limiting others. We can either choose blame or acceptance, to feel shame or feel blessed, to consent or to withdraw consent, to be unconscious or conscious, to manifest by default or by deliberation, to be fearful or loving. Everything is a choice to direct our life experiences.

I read somewhere that the purpose of fear is to save your life. Fear is meant to slap you into action, and take you out of danger to the center of your being where fear is transformed to love. Changing fear to love is easier said than done. It is one thing to say, "I love myself," and another to feel it in your bones and down into your cells. Loving is an inside job. Like building a muscle, living from the heart takes practice, and repetition. You might feel more pain before seeing any gains. Yet each time we don't neglect our hearts we start a revolution. When I let my heart speak, I awoke to my inner calling. When I opened the window to opportunity, I watched fear walk out the back door. Each new step became a dance. I gained confidence. And value. I appreciated.

You are what you perceive. Imagine it, embody it, and take action. When you stand firm in your truth and speak from your heart, you free yourself to heal. The body knows where to begin and what to do. It only asks, through its own language, that you pay attention. As one layer is healed another is revealed. Your frequency ripples out to touch others. The healing journey has no limits and no end. There is only the dance: stepping to the left and to the right, stepping back, and then moving forward again.

About the author

Rosanne Lindsay, ND, discovered her gifts as a healer through her own healing journey of reversing profound hypothyroidism by learning that we reclaim health and heal as individuals when we connect to nature and exercise our inherent freedom to choose.

Rosanne is a naturopath in Wisconsin. She holds graduate degrees from Trinity School of Natural Health in naturopathic medicine and the University of Chicago's School of Public Health in environmental health science. She serves as President of the National Health Freedom Coalition to preserve inherent rights and the freedom to choose.

Rosanne believes that reconnecting to Nature unleashes the healer within and that profound healing comes from taking profound measures. Her passion and mission are to guide others to drop the disease label and to reclaim their inheritance as healers.

Appendix I

Doc's Letter Showing Hypothyroidism Reversal

December 7, 2009

Dear Rosanne:

Here are the results from your last laboratory test(s):

Office visit on 12/07/2009

Component	Date	Value
TSH (ulU/mL)	12/07/2009	2.37
Free T4 (ng/dL)	12/07/2009	1.18
Free T3 (pg/mL)	12/07/2009	3.3

Comments:

All I can say is "Wow!" Nice numbers. I am really pleasantly surprised by these. In Europe they like to keep TSH between 2-3 in some countries, and your numbers are just right in terms of the other hormones. I am more than happy to let well enough alone with dosing for now and we can recheck in a few months (let me know, but I would say we could even wait til March or April with numbers this excellent).

If you have any questions regarding these results, please contact our office at ████████.

Sincerely,

████████, MD
Electronically signed.

Appendix II

BACK TO THE BASICS:

By incorporating the following traditional, inexpensive healing foods into your kitchen, you transfer the power of nature's remedies into your hands:

COCONUT OIL

- *2 Tablespoons a day added to smoothie or to oatmeal.*
- Promotes T4 to T3 conversion.
- Increases metabolism.
- Benefits heart, brain, nervous system, skin.
- Increases basal body temperature above 97°F.
- Promotes weight loss.
- Increases enzyme production.
- Functions as an antioxidant to reduce oxidative stress.
- Supports immunity when used in oil pulling by swishing 2 Tablespoons in mouth for 15 minutes daily. Spit in garbage when finished.

SEA SALT & KELP & SEA VEGETABLES

- *Add ½ teaspoon of sea salt per quart of water and shake to charge. Drink half your weight in ounces of water daily to hydrate.*
- Composed of trace minerals similar to the composition of the sea.

- Contains clay particles.
- Heals glands and nervous system.
- Preserves foods with antiseptic properties.
- Contains live magnesium.
- Contains iodine, about 60 micrograms per liter.
- Concentrates iodine to more than 30,000 times that found in seawater (Kelp, Nori, Dulse, Brown algae).
- Used in combination to balance hormonal deficiency (Irish Moss and Kelp).
- Increases metabolic rate, thyroid activity, and detoxification, and increase blood circulation and soothes inflamed tissues.
- Concentrates iodine for its antimicrobial and antioxidant properties.

BONE BROTH

- *In stock pot, add 3-4 lbs. beef marrow and knuckle bones, 2 Tbps. raw apple cider vinegar, 4 quarts filtered water, 3 celery stalks, 3 carrots, 2 onions, fresh cilantro, sea salt. Add water to cover bones. Bring to boil, reduce heat and simmer for 6-12 hours. Add cilantro in last 10 minutes. Let cool. Strain. Add sea salt to taste.*
- Heals leaky gut, supports digestion.
- Reduces joint pain and inflammation.
- Contains calcium, phosphorus, silicon, other trace minerals, glucosamine, bone marrow, collagen, glutamine, and healthy fats.
- Reduces inflammation and infection.
- Supports adrenals, bones, teeth.
- Promotes healthy hair and nails.

BLACK STRAP MOLASSES

- *Add 2 Tbsp. organic Black Strap molasses to oatmeal or smoothie.*
- Contains bioavailable minerals and vitamins such as iron, calcium, magnesium, selenium, and vitamin B6.
- Contains 50 percent RDA for calcium and 38 percent for magnesium in 5 Tbsp. as a bone booster.
- Contains 95 percent of RDA for iron in 5 Tbsp. as a blood booster against anemia.
- Relieves PMS.
- Stabilizes blood sugar levels.
- Enhances skin health.
- Improves depression, stress, and anxiety.
- Helps symptoms of ADHD.

LEMON

- *Squeeze half a lemon into 2 16 oz. glasses of water before breakfast to flush liver.*
- Aids digestion, stimulates biliary action.
- Stimulates, decongests, cleanses the liver.
- Aids high blood pressure, hardened arteries, and fragile blood vessels.
- Purifies blood.
- Targets parasites, pathogenic bacteria such as typhus and cholera.
- Dissolves crystals in joints, kidneys and bladder.

GARLIC

- *Best raw: 1-4 cloves of garlic (start with one). Put in glass of hot water, steep and dissolve overnight, filter and discard garlic, and drink the water.*[335]

- Contains sulfur iodine, and silica.
- Acts as natural antiseptic, disinfectant.
- Promotes glandular balance.
- Purifies blood.
- Aids joint stiffness.
- Increases gastric secretions and stomach wall motility.
- Stimulates appetite and digestion.

SPIRULINA OR GREENS POWDER

- *Add 1 Tbsp. to smoothie.*
- Superfood immune booster.
- Detoxifies metals such as lead, mercury.
- Detoxifies radiation and chemotherapy.
- Contains high amounts of iron, vitamin A, protein, B1, B2, B3, B6 magnesium, phosphorous and zinc.
- Balances blood sugar.
- Supports eye health.
- Promotes healthy skin.
- Promotes weight loss.
- Eases digestion and bowel movements.

II. AYURVEDIC MEDICINE:

GINGER

- *Warming food that harmonizes and promotes complete digestion.*
- Contains > 60 trace minerals, > 30 amino acids, > 500 enzymes.
- Acts as antiviral, antibacterial, antiparasitic.

- Supports immune system
- Relaxes muscles
- Enhances blood flow
- Regulates blood circulation
- Balances blood sugar
- Improves joint health
- Detoxifies
- Relaxes nerves
- Helps menstrual and muscle cramps, migraines, ganglia cysts, spastic colon, spastic bladder, pancreatitis, gallbladder spasms, stomach cramps, acid reflux, back pain, sinus pain, dizziness, urinary retention, incontinence, weight gain, chronic nausea, fatigue, anxiousness

BLACK PEPPER AND CAYENNE PEPPER

- *Spices that stimulate taste buds signaling the stomach to increase HCL secretions to improve digestion.*
- Releases blockages in throat chakra, thyroid, thymus, heart chakra, and CNS
- Stimulates glands
- Stops pain, warms body
- Cleanses and detoxifies
- Enhances digestion
- Improves mental alertness
- Acts as antiviral, antispasmodic
- Relieves sinus congestion and chronic bronchitis
- Increases effects and absorption of turmeric

ANISE SEED

- *Spicy aromatic used as a base in herbal teas, soups, sauces, breads, biscuits, cakes, and tastes like licorice*
- Soothes a sore throat
- Benefits asthma, bronchitis, cough
- Reduces intestinal gas, bloating, colic, nausea
- Promotes digestion
- Increases breast milk production

TURMERIC

- *Spice containing curcumin used in cooking and can be added to smoothie, or to make Golden Milk.*
- Fights inflammation.
- Improves digestion of fats and sugars
- Protects the heart
- Boosts brain power
- Remineralizes bone
- Detoxifies tissue
- Cleanses Candida overgrowth

III. CULINARY AND MEDICINAL HERBALISM

The ancient Egyptians, Indians, Chinese, Greeks, Romans and Native Americans were all herbalists. Through the Middle Ages, herbalism was preserved in the monasteries. Later, four main herbalists represent milestones in the history of herbalism that began with Greek surgeons Dioscorides and Galen who compiled herbals into the definitive *materia medica* texts that were used for the next 1500 years. In the 1500s, Paracelsus was an herbalist who introduced the "Doctrine of Signatures" showing how each herb has its own "sign" where its color, form, location, and scent identify its medicinal use. In the 1600s, Culpepper connected herbalism to astrology and the zodiac to determine what sign ruled over the body that needed care and matched it with the herb with the same astrological sign.

Today, herbalism continues to live through each of us that grow and use herbs in our own healing. Many people who work with herbs have discovered that if an herb grows wild in your yard, it is likely there because you need it's healing properties, so look down and do some digging. A few herbs used as food and medicine for thyroid disorders follow:

Ginseng – used as a spice it grows naturally in the mountains. It is sweet and a little bitter, known as a sexual tonic to enhance libido. Ginseng is energizing and a long-term stamina enhancer. Two grams per day is used in China where it is known as a panacea. Ninety-nine percent of ginseng comes from Korea, China, Canada, and America. The root is available dried or sliced and can be found as a root or as an herbal tea, tincture, or dietary supplement.

Gotu Kola – originates from the parsley family much like spinach. It is used as a cooked vegetable in Eastern parts of the world. Gotu kola can be juiced, steamed, pureed/spiced, hydrated and mixed with spinach. This herb benefits brain and nerve function, and increases memory, and prevents dementia. It increases blood vessel and collagen growth to improve the connective tissue of joints, ligaments, and tendons. It improves neuromuscular conditions and helps with strains, sprains, rashes, and skin. Leaves and stems can be harvested daily. Use fresh or dried. Cook and eat 30 grams per day or use as a powder.

Ashwagandha Root – an anti-oxidant, anti-inflammatory that supports metabolism. It can also lower stress and increase memory, energy and vitality. Ashwagandha also helps to improve sleep, adrenals, thyroid, and maintain proper nourishment of tissues, especially muscle and bone. Eight weeks on this herb as an extract or tincture can result in normalization of TSH, T4, and T3 in those with elevated TSH levels.[336] Contraindicated in pregnancy or nursing, or when taking anti-anxiety drugs. It grows naturally in the humid conditions of India, so find it locally for sale as a powder or tincture to use daily powdered in milk, or as a tincture or tea.

Calendula – a lymph tonic that also benefits the liver, nerves, skin, immune system, and blood. Calendula dispels chills/dampness, warms periphery and relaxes nerves. It is an antibiotic, antifungal, antiseptic, and anti-inflammatory for acute infections. According to herbalist, Matthew Wood, calendula also finds iodine in the body. The blossoms have been used to make medicine for thousands of years. Find and use as a tincture, tea, or in a salve for topical application.

Poke Root – a lymph tonic for autoimmune conditions. It is used for glandular and organ swellings, mastitis, intestinal cystitis, hard, swollen glands, tonsillitis, mumps, for pain in rheumatoid arthritis, and to move depressed functions. Pokeroot has anti-tumor effects and may benefit breast, ovarian, and prostate cancers that depend on hormones to grow. It interacts with T-cells to strengthen the immune system and is an antiviral, antifungal, and blood purifier. Use only minute amounts in a formula due to potency.

Oregon Grape Root – serves multiple purposes. It is a bitter to stimulate enzymes and the secretion of HCL in the stomach to improve digestion of fats, carbohydrates, and proteins. It assists a swollen liver, the lymphatic system, detoxifies, and improves waste removal though its laxative and diuretic effect. Oregon grape root contains berberine, which closes "tight junctions" of gut epithelial cells to reduce "leaky gut" according to Dr. Jeffrey

Dach. It down-regulates the inflammatory response in gut and brain[337] is a natural sedative/anti-depressant,[338] antifungal, and an antimicrobial. Not to be used in pregnancy. Use as a tincture in a formula, or drink as a tea, 4 oz., three times daily.

FOR HYPOTHYROIDISM

Black Walnut – (*Juglans nigra*) The hulls of black walnut contain tannins and juglone which are a source of iodine. Black walnut is used against parasites, yeast, and fungus, and to sooth a sour stomach. It can alleviate chronic constipation, diarrhea, acne and eczema, and hypothyroidism with poor liver metabolism. Not to be used in pregnancy. Use the hulls for tincture making; 5-10 drops, 3 to 4 times daily.

Bladderwrack – (*Fuscus vesiculosis*) used as the original source of iodine in the 19th century for thyroid disorders, bladderwrack is one of the most common types of seaweed found in the ocean. It has been used for centuries as an herbal remedy and culinary ingredient. This herb upregulates iodine processing hormones. Combined with Ashwagandha, it can stimulate thyroid hormone in some people with autoimmune disease. Since is improves metabolism, it helps with weight loss. Other benefits include improved vision, improved digestion, reduced inflammation, heart health, anti-aging, and cancer prevention. Contraindicated in hyperthyroidism. Use in an herbal formula.

Gum Guggul – or Guggul Myrrh extract (*Commiphora mukul*), stimulates the thyroid gland, enhances peripheral conversion of T4 to T3, aids in the reduction of cholesterol and inflammation. Do not take with prescription drugs, statins, anti-coagulants or St. John's Wort. Gum guggul can cause hypersensitivity reaction, rash and pruritus, therefore use in a formula, such as one with bladderwrack described below.

Blue Flag Root – (*Iris versicolor*) provides gentle glandular stimulation and detoxification. Use as an herbal tincture in a formula such as the one below with bladderwrack and gum guggul.

Bladderwrack, Gum guggul, and Blue Flag combined with Nettle leaf (*Urtica*), Triphala, and Bacopa (*B. monierri*) work synergistically to nourish the thyroid gland by enhancing its normal metabolic functions. [339] Individuals with high cholesterol, slow digestion, slow metabolism, or low body temperature may benefit from this herbal formulation. Note: Guggul and Iris are not recommended in pregnancy. Always seek the advice of a Master Herbalist or knowledgeable practitioner for herbal formulas. These people can provide guidance for any contraindications.

FOR HYPERTHYROIDISM

Lemon Balm – (*Melissa officinalis*) used primarily for anxiety, and insomnia. It also helps heart palpitations and high cholesterol. It calms the stomach, heart, and balances mood because it acts on the vagus nerve. Traditionally used to uplift the spirit and enhance memory, this herb was used to heal broken hearts and attract romantic love. Lemon balm can be used as a tincture, tea, or essential oil. Use as a single herb tincture, in combination, or as a tea.

Bungleweed – (*Lycopus virginicus*) a water-loving plant from the mint family used for overactive thyroid. Bugleweed influences the metabolism of iodine in the conversion of thyroid hormones. It may work to lower levels of TSH and binds to antibodies of the thyroid gland. It is used for symptoms of hyperthyroidism, which include anxiety, rapid heart rate, sensitivity to heat, anxiety, PMS, excessive sweating, and bulging eyes. It also controls nosebleeds and heavy menstruation. Do not take during pregnancy. This unusual sounding plant also goes by the names gypsywort, gypsyweed, and horehound.

Motherwort – (*Leonurus cardiaca*) also a member of the mint family, motherwort can help an overactive thyroid but does not depress normal thyroid function. As a cardiac tonic and nervine tonic, motherwort decreases muscle spasms and reduces high blood pressure due to stress and anxiety. Motherwort can slow heart palpitations, arrhythmias, nervous tachycardia, and reduce fat in blood. It improves mood, insomnia, and anxiety in those with hyperthyroidism, according to Herbalist Kathy Eich. Tincture is contraindicated in first 2 ½ trimesters of pregnancy. Motherwort is also called 'mother's herb' from the Greeks. It's Latin name, *leonurus,* means lion's tail, since it resembles one. Can be used in a formula with lemon balm and bugleweed for hyperthyroidism, depending on the individual.

V. TEAS AND JUICES

OAT STRAW TEA (*Avena sativa*):

- *Use in tea infusions, baths, and compresses for skin conditions from sunburn to rashes to eczema.*
- Nourishes and tonifies the nervous system at deepest level.
- Builds hair, skin, teeth, nails; high in calcium and silica.
- Benefits broken bones and combines with similar herbs like horsetail and comfrey.
- Calms and relaxes; high in B vitamins except B12.
- Acts on stress.

RED CLOVER BLOSSOM TEA (*TRIFOLIUM PRATENSE*):

- *Nourishing glandular remedy*
- Balances hormones; reduces symptoms of menopause.
- Fights respiratory infections, lowers mucus.
- Improves bone mineral density, high blood pressure, high cholesterol, and cardiovascular health.
- Detoxifies metals.
- Boosts immune system.

DANDELION LEAF, NETTLE LEAF, ATLANTIC KELP AND DULSE TEA:

- *Nutritious*
- Reverses radiation and liver damage.
- Acts on metabolism.
- Builds liver, clears excess waste; purifies blood.

CHAGA TEA:

- *"Black gold," ancient mushroom, grows on birch trees. Extract in alcohol, use in tincture for bioavailability.*
- Contains naturally occurring vanillin
- Modulates immune system; adaptogen.
- Balances blood sugar levels.
- Acts as antibacterial, antifungal, antiviral, antiparasitic, antiinflammatory, potent antioxidant.
- Aids in digestion
- Helps stomach pain, asthma, ulcers, bronchitis, liver, eczema, cancer, chronic fatigue, viral infections, stroke, rheumatoid arthritis, fibromyalgia.

CELERY JUICE

- *16 oz, celery twice a day. Use a masticating juicer for best results.*
- Restores hydrochloric acid in stomach naturally to promote digestion, cools digestive tract.
- Regenerates and strengthens bones; celery and bones are both twenty-three percent sodium. Contains vitamin K for calcium assimilation.
- Balances blood pH, purifies blood, neutralizes acidity, alkalinizes the gut.
- Relaxes nerves, natural laxative.

BEET JUICE (MIXED WITH CARROTS, AND APPLE)

- *Use organic beets and a masticating juicer.*
- Cleanses and detoxifies liver.
- Relieves pressure of hemorrhoids, reduces blood pressure.
- Improves circulation and sexual function, known as nature's Viagra.

V. EARTH AS MEDICINE

HEALING CLAY AS BENTONITE, MONTMORILLONITE, AND ILLITE INGESTED ORALLY. [340]

Mix 1 teaspoon in water. Take on empty stomach before bed or early morning. For more information see www.eatonsearth.org.

There is an adjustment period for beginners: Ingest 3 days. After the third day, abstain from clay use for four days. Then resume use for four days, and pause for the following three days. This method of use can be continued throughout the adjustment period which usually a few weeks.

- Is living earth, homeostatic, colloidal
- Catalyzes the removal of metals, toxins, foodborne pathogens, and radiation without removing trace minerals
- Kills many pathogens, removes others
- Fixes free oxygen in bloodstream and increases T-cell count
- Stimulates liver function, detoxifies liver
- Cleanses colon and balances bacterial species in intestine
- Improves digestive efficiency
- Reduces food sensitivities
- Stimulates circulation in body when used as a clay bath
- Strengthens general constitution to stimulate healing

INTERNAL CLAY PROTOCOL:—Internal ingestion of clay water (1 tsp. in water) can be split into 2 doses per day. Small amounts of clay water can be taken as often as every four hours if the individual can tolerate it, or at least twice daily for a period of no less than three days.

EXTERNAL CLAY PROTOCOL:—Use clay in a warm 20-minute bath. For acute conditions, 24-72 hours should pass before bathing in clay. This is because the bath will release some toxins into the lymphatic system for internal elimination and it is important to support the body's elimination systems during this 72-hour cycle.

VI. CANNABIS AND CANNABIDIOL (HEMP PLANT)

Cannabinoids in cannabis naturally occur in human breast milk. Our bodies and cell membranes contain cannabinoid receptors designed specifically to process cannabinoids such as tetrahydrocannibinol (THC), a primary active component of the cannabis plant. Cannabadiol (CBD) comes from the hemp plant, and is a phytocannabinoid with therapeutic properties for numerous conditions, especially neurodegenerative disorders. It also contains omega 3 fatty acids, vitamins, chlorophyll, amino acids and other nutrients. CBD acts as an anti-inflammatory, anticonvulsant, anti-oxidant, anti-emetic, anxiolytic and antipsychotic agent, and is therefore a potential medicine for neuro-inflammation, epilepsy, oxidative injury, vomiting and nausea, anxiety and schizophrenia.[341]

VII. Seeds, Nuts, Fruits

FOODS WITH THE HIGHEST SOURCES OF ABSORBABLE VITAMIN B17 (NATURAL LAETRILE).

Apricots including kernels and seeds; seeds from other fruits such as apples, cherries, peaches, prunes, plums, and pears; lima beans, fava beans, wheatgrass, almonds, raspberries, elderberries, strawberries, blackberries, blueberries, buckwheat sorghum, barley, millet, cashews, macadamia nuts, and bean sprouts.

How easy to add a few nuts or berries to cereal, snacks, or salads. And the health benefits show up as increased vitality, clear skin, strong nails and hair, improved digestion, clear thinking, and balanced moods.

Appendix III

VITAMIN D SUPPLEMENTATION: GOOD OR BAD?

In all autoimmune disease, including Hashimoto's and Graves' disease, vitamin D is found to be lacking. Current belief holds that D-deficiency is a cause of disease even though evidence shows that D-deficiency is the result of disease. Understanding this difference is critical.

Vitamin D is not a vitamin at all; it is similar to cortisol and testosterone, making it a steroid hormone. As a steroid hormone, D works within a self-regulating system to bind to its own vitamin D-binding protein receptor on every cell. Why is this important?

Vitamin D is biphasic. It functions like an adaptogen. This means vitamin D can adapt itself as both an active form, 1,25-D, and an inactive form, 25-D, depending on how the body intends to use it. "Homeostatic regulation" means that our hormones modulate immunity directed by the body, not the doctor. Like our glands, hormones work in cooperation with other hormones, substrates, ligands, enzymes, bacteria, minerals, receptor sites, and energy. Under most conditions, the active form of vitamin D acts as the "on" switch to upregulate immunity, while the inactive form acts as the "off" switch to downregulate immunity.

Without a clear appreciation of D as a self-regulator, most

allopathic and natural doctors, alike, rush to supplement people identified as having "low" D levels. Not only do medical doctors make a mistake in measuring the inactive form, they also prescribe D2, an irradiated plant-based form that is not fat soluble like D3, and therefore not absorbed. The popular prescription Vitamin D2, Drisdol, carries the following warning (among others):

> Dosage levels must be individualized and great care exercised to prevent serious toxic effects. In Vitamin D resistant rickets the range between therapeutic and toxic doses is narrow.

All doctors who tout supplementation fail to consider an alternative hypothesis—that D deficiency is a result of the inflammatory disease process, not the cause.[342]

Research shows that reduced levels of vitamin D can result from chronic infection, or Th1 illnesses. The infection stems from intracellular bacteria, or Th1 pathogens, that dysregulate vitamin D metabolism by causing vitamin D receptor dysfunction within phagocytes.[343] Simply put, disease is caused by our own pleomorphic bacteria that get inside the cells to block the production of energy by our mitochondria.

Supplementing with active D form of the hormone can have a biphasic effect. At low concentrations it can be stimulating, while at higher levels it can become ineffective and problematic. In the same way that autoimmune disease responds to corticosteroid (Prednisone) treatment, vitamin D can temporarily reduce symptoms of disease. However long-term use can dramatically increase the odds of disease relapse.

Supplementing with excess vitamin D3 undercuts our self-regulating feedback system. The thyroid gland is typically the first victim of excess D because this active steroid hormone will park in the thyroid receptor site to block active thyroid hormone.

Remember, a poorly functioning thyroid is often the result of T4 hormone not converting into the bioactive hormone, T3. Instead, it converts into the inactive rT3 hormone. As rT3 levels increase, T3 levels fall causing hypothyroidism. Metabolism and body temp decrease and various enzymes fail to function properly. In addition, elevated cortisol due to adrenal dysfunction can contribute to this faulty conversion.

The body selects for inactive thyroid hormone at the receptor site in the same way it selects for inactive vitamin D. When thyroid autoantibodies are present, the receptor for vitamin D changes to select for the inactive form of vitamin D. In other words, both thyroid hormone and vitamin D hormone downregulate metabolism in response to inflammation caused by a shift in our microbes at the level of the gut across different cultural groups.[344]

Appendix IV

A healthy body frequency has been measured to be between 62 and 72 MHz. Disease begins around 58 MHz. Candida overgrowth starts at 55 MHz, a natural response to toxic overload. Epstein-Barr Virus is receptive at 52 MHz, cancer at 42 MHz, and death starts at 25 MHz.[345]

<u>IDEAL HUMAN BODY FREQUENCIES:</u>

Genius Brain Frequency: 80-82 MHz

Brain Frequency Range: 72-90 MHz

Normal Brain Frequency: 72 MHz

Human Body: 62-78 MHz

Human Body: from Neck up : 72-78 MHz

Human Body: from Neck down: 60-68 MHz

Thyroid and Parathyroid glands: 62-68 MHz

Thymus Gland: 65-68 MHz

Heart: 67-70 MHz

Lungs: 58-65 MHz

Liver: 55-60 MHz

ENDNOTES

1   Wang, Clifford, and Lawrence M. Crapo. "The Epidemiology Of Thyroid Disease And Implications For Screening." *Endocrinology and Metabolism Clinics of North America* 26, no. 1 (March 1997): 189-218. doi:10.1016/S0889-8529(05)70240-1.

2   Mark P. J. Vanderpump; The epidemiology of thyroid disease. *Br Med Bull* 2011; 99 (1): 39-51. doi: 10.1093/bmb/ldr030.

3   Louis, Berman. *The glands regulating personality a study of the glands of internal secretion in relation to the types of human nature.* New York, NY: Macmillan, 1921.

4   Burd-Sharps, S. Lewis, K, et al., The Measure of America, American Human Development Report | 2008-2009, A joint publication of the Social Science Research Council and Columbia, University Press, July 16, 2008.

5   Starfield, B. "Is US Health Really the Best in the World?" JAMA: The Journal of the American Medical Association 284, no. 4 (2000): 483-85. doi:10.1001/jama.284.4.483.

6   James, John T. "A New, Evidence-based Estimate of Patient Harms Associated with Hospital Care." *Journal of Patient Safety* 9.3 (2013): 122-28. Web. <http://journals.lww.com/

journalpatientsafety/Fulltext/2013/09000/A_New,_Evidence_
based_Estimate_of_Patient_Harms.2.aspx>.

7   Andel, C., S. L. Davidow, M. Hollander, and D. A. Moreno.
       "The Economics of Health Care Quality and Medical Errors."
       J Health Care Finance 39.1 (2012): 39-50. Pubmed, 2012. Web.
       <https://www.ncbi.nlm.nih.gov/pubmed/23155743>.

8   Lauden, Aron, and Danielle Johnson. U.S. Health in
       International Perspective Shorter Lives, Poorer Health. Report.
       January 2013. https://www.iom.edu/~/media/Files/Report%20
       Files/2013/US-Health-International-Perspective/USHealth_
       Intl_PerspectiveRB.pdf.

9   Schoen, Davis Stremikis Squires. EXECUTIVE SUMMARY—
       Mirror, Mirror on the Wall: How the Performance of the U.S.
       Health Care System Compares Internationally, 2014 Update,
       June 2014.

10   Davis, Karen, Kristof Stremikis, David Squires, and Cathy
       Schoen. *2014 Update Mirror Mirror On The Wall*. Rep.
       Commonwealth Fund, June 2014. Web. <http://www.common-
       wealthfund.org/~/media/files/publications/fund-report/2014/
       jun/1755_davis_mirror_mirror_2014.pdf>.

11   Makary, Martin A., and Michael Daniel. "Medical error—the
       third leading cause of death in the US." *Bmj* 353 (May 03, 2016):
       I2139. doi:10.1136/bmj.i2139.

12   Kantor, Elizabeth D. et al. "Trends in Prescription Drug Use
       Among Adults in the United States From 1999-2012." *Jama*
       314.17 (2015): 1818. Web.

13   *The Hidden Side of Clinical Trails*. By Sile Lane. Perf. Sile Lane.
       The Hidden Side of Clinical Trails. TedX, 19 Oct. 2016. Web. <
       https://www.youtube.com/watch?v=-RXrGLolgEc>.

14   C. Glenn Begley & Lee M. Ellis, Nature 483, 531–533, Drug development: Raise standards for preclinical cancer research, 29 March 2012.

15   Jones, Hardin B. "Section Of Biology: Demographic Consideration Of The Cancer Problem*." *Transactions of the New York Academy of Sciences* 18.4 Series II (1956): 298-333. Web. <https://www.researchgate.net/publication/10254549_Demographic_consideration_of_the_cancer_problem>.

16   The Death of Blind Faith. Directed by Joseph Mercola. Most Astonishing Health Disaster of the 20th Century. July 30, july. https://www.youtube.com/watch?v=FPI7zdGdqo4.

17   Ferrie, Helke. "ALTERNATIVE MEDICINE TAKES ON CANCER – AND WINS." *Vitality*, 1 Nov. 2010. http://vitalitymagazine.com/article/alternative-medicine-takes-on-cancer-and-wins/.

18   Davies, P C W, and C H Lineweaver. "Cancer tumors as Metazoa 1.0: tapping genes of ancient ancestors." *Physical Biology*, vol. 8, no. 1, Jan. 2011, p. 015001., doi:10.1088/1478-3975/8/1/015001.

19   Brownstein, David, M.D. Lecture, Overcoming Hypothyroidism, ZRT Laboratory's Webinar, 2009. Accessed 2009. http://www.purebodysolutions.com/mm5/graphics/PDF/ZRT/OvercomingHypothyroidismLectureSlides.pdf.

20   Wang, Clifford, and Lawrence M. Crapo. "The Epidemiology Of Thyroid Disease And Implications For Screening." *Endocrinology and Metabolism Clinics of North America* 26, no. 1 (March 1997): 189-218. doi:10.1016/S0889-8529(05)70240-1.

21   Esselborn-Krumbiegel, Helga. *Hermann Hesse, Der Steppenwolf: Interpretation.* Oldenbourg, 1998.

22   Weinhold, Bob. "Epigenetics: The Science of Change."

Environmental Health Perspectives 114.3 (2006): n. pag. Web. <https://www.ncbi.nlm.nih.gov/pmc/articles/PMC1392256/>.

23   Moss, Robert. "There Is One Direction in Which Space Is Open to Us." Web log post. *The Robert Moss Blog.* Robert Moss, 02 May 2016. Web. <http://mossdreams.blogspot.com/2016/05/there-is-one-direction-in-which-space.html?spref=fb>.

24   Harach H.R et al. Thyroid carcinoma and thyroiditis in an endemic goitre region before and after iodine prophylaxis. Acta Endocrinol (Copenh) 1985;108:55–60. [PubMed]

25   Pope, C. A., Aruni Bhatnagar, James McCracken, and Wesley T Abplanalp. "Exposure to Fine Particulate Air Pollution Is Associated with Endothelial Injury and Systemic Inflammation." *Circulation Research.* Circres.ahajournals.org, 25 Oct. 2016. Web. <http://circres.ahajournals.org/content/early/2016/10/19/CIRCRESAHA.116.309279>.

26   Tomljenovic , L., & Shaw, C. A. (2012). Mechanisms of aluminum adjuvant toxicity and autoimmunity in pediatric populations. *Lupus,2*, 223-30. doi:10.1177/0961203311430221

27   Mold, Matthew, Ducas Umar, Andrew King, and Christopher Exley. "Aluminium in brain tissue in Autism." *Journal of Trace Elements in Medicine and Biology*46 (March2018):76-82. http://www.sciencedirect.com/science/article/pii/S0946672X17308763.

28   Mirza, Ambreen, Anrew King, and Christopher Exley. "Aluminium in brain tissue in familial Alzheimer's disease." *Aluminium in brain tissue in familial Alzheimer's disease*40 (March2017):30-36. http://www.sciencedirect.com/science/article/pii/S0946672X16303777.

29   Vera-Lastra, O. et al. (2013). Autoimmune/inflammatory syndrome induced by adjuvants (Shoenfeld's syndrome): clinical and

immunological spectrum. *Expert Review of Clinical Immunology,* *9*(4), 361-373. doi:10.1586/eci.13.2

30   Mirza, A., King, A., Troakes, C., & Exley, C. (2107). Aluminium in brain tissue in familial Alzheimer's disease. *Journal of Trace Elements in Medicine and Biology,40*, 30-6. http://dx.doi.org/10.1016/j.jtemb.2016.12.001

31   Exley, C., PhD. (2018, June 19). Silicon-rich water and aluminium detoxification [E-mail to the author]. https://www.hippocraticpost.com/?s=Exley

32   Aceves, Carmen et al. "The Extrathyronine Actions of Iodine as Antioxidant, Apoptotic, and Differentiation Factor in Various Tissues." *Thyroid* 23.8 (2013): 938-46. Web. <https://www.ncbi.nlm.nih.gov/pmc/articles/PMC3752513/>.

33   William, Anthony. *Medical Medium: Secrets behind Chronic and Mystery Illness and How to Finally Heal.* N.p.: n.p., n.d. *Goop.com.* Web. <http://goop.com/the-medical-medium-and-whats-potentially-at-the-root-of-medical-mysteries/>.

34   Young, L. S., & Rickinson, A. B. (2004). Epstein–Barr virus: 40 years on. *Nature Reviews Cancer,4*, 757-68. doi:10.1038/nrc1452.

35   Gregerman RI and Solomon N. "Acceleration of thyroxine and triiodothyronine turnover during bacterial pulmonary infection and fever: implications for the functional state of the thyroid during stress and senescence." J Clin Endocr $ Metab, 1967; 27:93.

36   Wang, H., Lee, I. S., Braun, C., & Enck, P. (2016). Effect of Probiotics on Central Nervous System Functions in Animals and Humans: A Systematic Review. *J Neurogastroenterol Motil., 30* (22), 4th ser., 589-605. Retrieved from https://www.ncbi.nlm.nih.gov/pubmed/27413138.

37   Möhle, Mattei, and Heimesaat et al. "Ly6Chi Monocytes Provide a Link between Antibiotic-Induced Changes in Gut Microbiota and Adult Hippocampal Neurogenesis." *Cell Reports*, 2016 DOI:10.1016/j.celrep.2016.04.074

38   Natasha DeLeon-Rodriguez, et al., "Microbiome of the upper troposphere: Species composition and prevalence, effects of tropical storms, and atmospheric implications," Proceedings of the National Academy of Sciences (2013): www.pnas.org/cgi/doi/10.1073/pnas.1212089110.

39   Gatti, Antonietta., (2017). New Quality-Control Investigations on Vaccines: Microand Nanocontamination. *International Journal of Vaccines and Vaccination,4*(1). Retrieved January 27, 2017, from http://medcraveonline.com/IJVV/IJVV-04-00072.pdf

40   Carley, Rebecca, MD. "I Just Never Knew Auto-antibodies Were Such a Drag." *Vaccines*. Vaccines by the Outliers, 18 Aug. 2016. Web. 20 Aug. 2016. <https://vaccinesbytheoutliers.wordpress.com/2016/08/18/i-just-never-knew-auto-antibodies-were-such-a-drag/>.

41   Benias, Petros C. et al. "Structure and Distribution of an Unrecognized Interstitium in Human Tissues." *Scientific Reports*, vol. 8, no. 1, 2018, doi:10.1038/s41598-018-23062-6.

42   Cell Press. "Antibodies are not required for immunity against some viruses." ScienceDaily. ScienceDaily, 1 March 2012. <www.sciencedaily.com/releases/2012/03/120301143426.htm>

43   Huang, Yongsheng et al. "Temporal Dynamics of Host Molecular Responses Differentiate Symptomatic and Asymptomatic Influenza A Infection." *PLoS Genetics* 7, no. 8 (2011). doi:10.1371/journal.pgen.1002234.

44   Ibid. Huang et al. "Temporal Dynamics of Host Molecular Responses Differentiate Symptomatic and Asymptomatic Influenza A Infection."

45   Sensor, David. Et al. *Epidemiologic Basis for Eradication of Measles in 1967.* Pubic Health Reports, 1969, pp. 253–256.

46   Serres, Gaston De. Et al. "Largest Measles Epidemic in North America in a Decade—Quebec, Canada, 2011: Contribution of Susceptibility, Serendipity, and Superspreading Events." *The Journal of Infectious Diseases*, vol. 207, no. 6, 2012, pp. 990–998., doi:10.1093/infdis/jis923.

47   Lund GA. Et al. "The molecular length of measles virus RNA and the structural organization of measles nucleocapsids." *J Gen Virol.* 1984 Sep;65 (Pt 9):1535–42.

48   Alison M. Hixon, Guixia Yu, J. Smith Leser, Shigeo Yagi, Penny Clarke, Charles Y. Chiu, Kenneth L. Tyler. "A mouse model of paralytic myelitis caused by enterovirus D68." *PLOS Pathogens*, 2017; 13 (2): e1006199 DOI: 10.1371/journal.ppat.1006199.

49   Johnson, Christine. "There Is No HIV Virus, An interview with Dr Eleni Papadopulos-Eleopulos By Christine Johnson from Continuum Autumn 1997." There is no HIV virus: an interview with Dr E. Papadopulos (1997). Accessed February 19, 2017. http://www.ourcivilisation.com/aids/hivexist/.

50   Doshi, Peter, PhD. "Influenza: Marketing Vaccines by Marketing Disease." *BMJ* 346 (2013): F3037.

51   Hqanon. "Anti-Vaxxer Biologist Stefan Lanka Bets Over $100K Measles Isn't A Virus; He Wins In German Federal Supreme Court." AnonHQ. January 21, 2017. http://anonhq.com/anti-vaxxer-biologist-stefan-lanka-bets-100k-measles-isnt-virus-wins-german-federal-supreme-court/.

52   OLG Stuttgart. *OLG Stuttgart Urteil vom 16.2.2016, 12 U 63/15.* Feb. 2016. http://lrbw.juris.de/cgi-bin/laender_rechtsprechung/document.py?Gericht=bw&GerichtAuswahl=Oberlandesgerichte&Art=en&sid=46bf3db2df690aba6e4874acafaf45b6&nr=20705&pos=0&anz=1. Quote Paragraph 20.

53   Søgaard, Mette, et al. "Hypothyroidism and Hyperthyroidism and Breast Cancer Risk: A Nationwide Cohort Study." *Eur J Endocrinol European Journal of Endocrinology* 174.4 (2016): 409-14. Web. <http://www.eje-online.org/content/174/4/409.abstract>.

54   Villoldo, Alberto. *Shaman, healer, sage: how to heal yourself and others with the energy medicine of the Americas.* Bantam, 2001.

55   Wood, Lawrence C., David S. Cooper, and E. Chester. Ridgway. *Your Thyroid: A Home Reference.* Boston: Houghton Mifflin, 1982.

56   A.D.A.M., and Harvey Simon, M.D. "Hypothyroidism." Hypothyroidism - In Depth Report." March 30, 2014. http://www.nytimes.com/health/guides/disease/hypothyroidism/background.html

57   Shomon, Mary J. *Living Well with Hypothyroidism: What Your Doctor Doesn't Tell You ... That You Need to Know.* New York: HarperResource, 2005. Print.

58   Pearce, Elizabeth N. "Iodine in Pregnancy: Is Salt Iodization Enough?" *The Journal of Clinical Endocrinology & Metabolism* 93.7 (2008): 2466-468.

59   Wang, Clifford, and Lawrence M. Crapo. "The Epidemiology Of Thyroid Disease And Implications For Screening." *Endocrinology and Metabolism Clinics of North America* 26, no. 1 (March 1997): 189-218. doi:10.1016/S0889-8529(05)70240-1.

60 Furszyfer J, Kurland LT, Woolner LB, *et al. "Hashimoto's thyroiditis in Olmsted County, Minnesota, 1935 through 1967."* May Clin Proc, 1970; 45:586-596.

61 Santin, Ana Paula, and Tania Weber Furlanetto. "Role of Estrogen in Thyroid Function and Growth Regulation." *Journal of Thyroid Research.* SAGE-Hindawi Access to Research, n.d. Web. 01 Jan. 2016.

62 D'Adamo, Peter, and Catherine Whitney. *Eat Right 4 (for) Your Type: The Individualized Diet Solution to Staying Healthy, Living Longer & Achieving Your Ideal Weight: 4 Blood Types, 4 Diets.* New York: G.P. Putnam's Sons, 1996. Print.

63 "The Thyroid Gland." *The Thyroid Gland - Iodine Source - Your Resource for Detoxified Iodine.*, ww.iodinesource.com/ThyroidGland.php#ThyroidGland.

64 Cashman, Leo. "Dental Amalgam Fillings: The Number One Source of Mercury Exposure Exceeds Government Health Standards - DAMS - Dental Amalgam Mercury Solutions." *DAMS.* Dental Amalgam Mercury Solutions, 2016. Web. <http://amalgam.org/education/scientific-evidenceresearch/dental-amalgam-fillings-number-one-source-mercury-exposure-exceeds-government-health-standards/>.

65 Centanni, Marco, Lucilla Gargano, and Gianluca Canettieri. "Thyroxine in Goiter, Helicobacter Pylori Infection, and Chronic Gastritis." *New England Journal of Medicine N Engl J Med* 354.17 (2006): 1787-795.

66 Singer, P. A., D. S. Cooper, E. G. Levy, P. W. Ladenson, L. E. Braverman, et al. "Treatment Guidelines for Patients With Hyperthyroidism and Hypothyroidism." *JAMA: The Journal of the American Medical Association* 273, no. 10 (March 08, 1995): 808-12. doi:10.1001/jama.1995.03520340064038.

67   Patel, H., Stalcup et al.: "The effect of excipients on the stability of levothyroxine sodium pentahydrate tablets." *Int. J. Pharm.*, 264(1-2): 35-43, 2003.

68   Alliance for Natural Health, 2011, August 9., Can My Doctor Get Into Big Legal Trouble by Offering Natural Health Treatments? Retrieved from https://www.sott.net/article/234931-Can-My-Doctor-Get-Into-Big-Legal-Trouble-by-Offering-Natural-Health-Treatments

69   Walsh, John P. et al. "Combined Thyroxine/Liothyronine Treatment Does Not Improve Well-Being, Quality of Life, or Cognitive Function Compared to Thyroxine Alone: A Randomized Controlled Trial in Patients with Primary Hypothyroidism." *The Journal of Clinical Endocrinology & Metabolism* 88.10 (2003): 4543-550.

70   Clyde, Patrick W., et al. "Combined Levothyroxine Plus Liothyronine Compared With Levothyroxine Alone in Primary Hypothyroidism." *JAMA* 290.22 (2003): 2952.

71   Sawka, A. M., H. C. et al. "Does a Combination Regimen of Thyroxine (T 4) and 3,5,3⊠-Triiodothyronine Improve Depressive Symptoms Better Than T 4 Alone in Patients with Hypothyroidism? Results of a Double-Blind, Randomized, Controlled Trial." *The Journal of Clinical Endocrinology & Metabolism* 88.10 (2003): 4551-555.

72   Rodriguez, Tom, et al. "Substitution Of Liothyronine At A 1:5 Ratio For A Portion Of Levothyroxine: Effect On Fatigue, Symptoms Of Depression, And Working Memory Versus Treatment With Levothyroxine Alone." *Endocrine Practice* 11.4 (2005): 223-33.

73   Cooper DS. "*Treatment of Thyrotoxicosis.*" *In:* Werner & Ingbar's

The Thyroid. Braverman LE and Utiger RD, editors. Lippincott Williams & Wilkins, 2000; 691-715.

74   Wartofsky L. *"Has the use of antithyroid drugs for Graves' disease become obsolete?"* Thyroid, 1993; 3:335-344.

75   Cooper DS. "Treatment of Thyrotoxicosis" *In:* Werner & Ingbar's The Thyroid. Braverman LE and Utiger RD, editors. Lippincott Williams & Wilkins, 2000; 691-715.

76   Williams KV, Nayak S, Becker D, et al. "Fifty years of experience with propylthiouracil-associated hepatotoxicity: What have we learned?" *J Clin Endocr & Metab*, 1997; 82:1727-1733.

77   Abraham, G.E. "The Safe and Effective Implementation of Orthoiodosupplementation In Medical Practice."

78   Ron, Elaine. "Thyroid Cancer Incidence Among People Living In Areas Contaminated By Radiation From The Chernobyl Accident." *Health Physics* 93, no. 5 (November 2007): 502-11. doi:10.1097/01.hp.0000279018.93081.29.

79   Ricarte-Filho, Julio C. et al. "Identification of kinase fusion oncogenes in post-Chernobyl radiation-induced thyroid cancers." *Journal of Clinical Investigation* 123, no. 11 (2013): 4935-944. doi:10.1172/jci69766.

80   Festen C, Otten BJ, van de Kaa CA. Follicular adenoma of the thyroid gland in children. *Eur J Pediatr Surg*. Oct 1995;5(5):262-4. [Medline]

81   Vane D, King DR, Boles ET Jr. Secondary thyroid neoplasms in pediatric cancer patients: increased risk with improved survival. *J Pediatr Surg*. Dec 1984;19(6):855-60. [Medline].

82   Mary Felber, Fredric J. Burns and Seymour J. Garte, Amplification of the c-myc Oncogene in Radiation-Induced Rat

Skin Tumors as a Function of Linear Energy Transfer and Dose, *Radiation Research*, Vol. 131, No. 3 (Sep., 1992), pp. 297-301 (article consists of 5 pages), Published by: Radiation Research Society [Abstract]

83   Sklar C, Whitton J, Mertens A, et al. Abnormalities of the thyroid in survivors of Hodgkin's disease: data from the Childhood Cancer Survivor Study. *J Clin Endocrinol Metab*. Sep 2000;85(9):3227-32. [Medline].

84   Yoskovitch A, Laberge JM, Rodd C, et al. Cystic thyroid lesions in children. *J Pediatr Surg*. Jun 1998;33(6):866-70. [Medline].

85   Garcia CJ, Daneman A, Thorner P, et al. Sonography of multinodular thyroid gland in children and adolescents. *Am J Dis Child*. 1992 Jul. 146(7):811-6.

86   Gerber, Mark E., MD. "Pediatric Thyroid Cancer." *Medscape*. Medscape, 30 Apr. 2015. Web. <http://emedicine.medscape.com/article/853737-overview>.

87   V B Nesterenko, A V Nesterenko, V I Babenko, T V Yerkovich, I V Babenko. "Reducing the 137Cs-load in the organism of "Chernobyl" children with apple-pectin." *Swiss Med Wkly*. 2004 Jan 10;134(1-2):24-7. PMID: 14745664

88   G S Bandazhevskaya et al. "Relationship between caesium (137Cs) load, cardiovascular symptoms, and source of food in 'Chernobyl' children — preliminary observations after intake of oral apple pectin." *Swiss Med Wkly*. 2004 Dec 18;134(49-50):725-9. PMID: 15635491

89   V S Kalistratova et al. "Study of the effect of a food additive Medetopect on metabolic kinetics of transuranic radionuclides in animal body." *Radiats Biol Radioecol*. 1998 Jan-Feb;38(1):35-41. PMID: 9606404

90   Abraham, G.E. "The Safe and Effective Implementation of Orthoiodosupplementation In Medical Practice."

91   Abraham, G.E. "The Safe and Effective Implementation of Orthoiodosupplementation In Medical Practice."

92   Dodds, Jean. "The Hidden Signs of Hypothyroidism You Don't Want to Miss." Healthy Pets with Dr. Karen Becker. July 19, 2011. http://healthypets.mercola.com/sites/healthypets/archive/2011/07/19/yes-you-can-get-a-oneyear-heads-up-that-your-dog-is-hypothyroid.aspx.

93   Lougheed, Barbara. "TSH Levels Fluctuate and Often Do Not Reflect Thyroid Levels." TiredThyroid.com. 2011-14. http://tiredthyroid.com/tsh.html.

94   Canaris, G. J. "The Colorado Thyroid Disease Prevalence Study." *Archives of Internal Medicine* 160, no. 4 (February 28, 2000): 526-34. doi:10.1001/archinte.160.4.526

95   Scobbo RR, VonDohlen TW, Hassan M, Islam S. Serum TSH variability in normal individuals: the influence of time of sample collection. W V Med J. 2004 Jul-Aug;100(4):138-42. http://www.ncbi.nlm.nih.gov/pubmed/15471172

96   Van Den Beld et al. "Reverse T3 Is the Best Measurement of Thyroid Tissue Levels." *Journal of Clinical Endocrinology & Metabolism* 90, no. 12, 6403-409.

97   Shomon, Mary. "Rethinking the TSH Test: An Interview with David Derry, M.D., Ph.D.The History of Thyroid Testing, Why the TSH Test Needs to Be Abandoned, and the Return to Symptoms-Based Thyroid Diagnosis and Treatment - Articles / FAQs." *Rethinking the TSH Test: An Interview with David Derry, M.D., Ph.D.The History of Thyroid Testing, Why the TSH Test Needs to Be Abandoned, and the Return to Symptoms-Based*

Thyroid Diagnosis and Treatment - Articles / FAQs. Thyroid-info. com, 13 Nov. 2015.

98   Mariano, Romeo. "The Usefulness of TSH | DEFINITIVE MIND." DEFINITIVE MIND. July 24, 2010. Accessed 2014. http://www.definitivemind.com/2010/07/24/ the-usefulness-of-tsh/.

99   Zimmermann, M., P. Adou, T. Torresani, C. Zeder, and R. Hurrell. "Iron Supplementation in Goitrous, Iron-deficient Children Improves Their Response to Oral Iodized Oil." *European Journal of Endocrinology* 142.3 (2000): 217-23.

100   Centanni, Marco, Lucilla Gargano, and Gianluca Canettieri. "Thyroxine in Goiter, Helicobacter Pylori Infection, and Chronic Gastritis." *New England Journal of Medicine N Engl J Med* 354.17 (2006): 1787-795.

101   Brownstein, David. *Drugs That Don't Work and Natural Therapies That Do!* West Bloomfield, MI: Medical Alternatives, 2007.

102   Prasad, Vinay, Andrae Vandross, Caitlin Toomy, Michael Cheung et al. "A Decade of Reversal: An Analysis of 146 Contraindicated Medical Practices." *Mayo Clinic Proceedings* 88. no. 8 (2013): 790-98.

103   Angell, M. (2009, January 15). Drug Companies & Doctors: A Story of Corruption. *The New York Review of Books.* Retrieved from http://www.nybooks.com/articles/2009/01/15/ drug-companies-doctorsa-story-of-corruption/.

104   Ioannidis, John P. A. "Why Most Published Research Findings Are False."*PLoS Med PLoS Medicine* 2.8 (2005): n. pag. PLoS. org, 30 Aug. 2005. Web. <http://journals.plos.org/plosmedicine/ article?id=10.1371/journal.pmed.0020124>.

105   Ioannidis, John P. A. "An Epidemic of False Claims." *Sci Am*

Scientific American 304.6 (2011): 16. Web. <http://www.scientificamerican.com/article/an-epidemic-of-false-claims/>.

106   Korch, Christopher. "DNA Profiling Analysis of Endometrial and Ovarian Cell Lines Reveals Misidentification, Redundancy and Contamination." *DNA Profiling Analysis of Endometrial and Ovarian Cell Lines Reveals Misidentification, Redundancy and Contamination*, vol. 127, no. 1, Oct. 2012, pp. 241–248., doi:doi.org/10.1016/j.ygyno.2012.06.017.

107   Neimark, J. "Line of attack." *Science*, vol. 347, no. 6225, 27 Feb. 2015, pp. 938–40., doi:10.1126/science.347.6225.938.

108   Grant, Bob. "Elsevier Published 6 Fake Journals." *The Scientist*. The Scientist.com, 07 May 2009. Web. <http://www.the-scientist.com/?articles.view/articleNo/27383/title/Elsevier-published-6-fake-journals/>.

109   Rector-Page, Linda G. *Diets for Healthy Healing: Dr. Linda Page's Natural Solutions to America's Biggest Health Problems: Includes Recipes, Exercises and More*. Del Rey Oaks, CA: Healthy Healing, 2005. P. 205.

110   Sircus, Mark, Ac., OMD. "Iodine and Chelation." *AFH LIBRARY -*. International Medical Veritas Association, 2007. Web. 30 Jan. 2016. <http://www.alkalizeforhealth.net/Liodine2.htm>.

111   Abraham, Gary E., M.D., and J. D. Flechas, M.D. "Evidence of Defective Cellular Oxidation and Organification of Iodide in a Female with Fibromyalgia and Chronic Fatigue." *The Original Alchemist Special Edition*: 194-99. http://www.optimox.com/pics/Iodine/pdfs/IOD20.pdf.

112   Sircus, Mark. "Iodine Treats and Prevents Cancer." *Dr. Sircus*, 10 May 2017, drsircus.com/iodine/iodine-treats-prevents-cancer/.

113   Sircus, Mark. "Iodine, Metabolism and Oxygen." *Dr. Sircus*, Http://Drsircus.com, 14 July 2017, drsircus.com/iodine/ iodine-metabolism-oxygen/.

114   Abraham, G.E., Flechas, J.D., & Hakala, J.C. (2002). Orthoiodosupplementation: Iodine sufficiency of the whole human body. The Original Internist, 9(4), 30-41. Retrieved from https://www.hakalalabs.com/media/wysiwyg/pdf_resources/ Abraham_OI_Dec02.pdf.

115   Abraham, G.E., "The Wolff-Chaikoff Effect: Crying Wolf?" *The Original Internist*, 12(3):112-118, 2005

116   Wartofsky L, Ransil BJ, and Ingbar SH. "Inhibition by iodine of the release of thyroxine from the thyroid glands of patients with thyrotoxicosis." *J Clin Invest*, 1970; 49: 78-86.

117   Wolff J and Chaikoff IL. "Plasma inorganic iodide as a homeostatic regulator of thyroid function." J Biol Chem, 1948:174: 555-564.

118   WHO. *Urinary Iodine Concentrations for Determining Iodine Status in Populations.* 2013.http://apps.who.int/iris/bitstream/10665/85972/1/WHO_NMH_NHD_EPG_13.1_eng. pdf?ua=1.

119   Abraham, G.E. "The Safe and Effective Implementation of Orthoiodosupplementation In Medical Practice."

120   Cousens, Gabriel. "Iodine – The Universal & Holistic Super Mineral." *Treeoflifecenterus.com*, 26 Dec. 2017, treeoflifecenterus. com/blog-posts-by-gabriel-cousens-m-d-iodine-96-the-universal-holistic-super-mineral-2/.

121   Bernecker C. *"Intermittent therapy with potassium iodide in chronic obstructive disease of the airways.."* Acta Allerg, 1969;24:171.

122   Hercheimer H. *"Effect of iodide treatment on thyroid function."* NEJM, 1977; 297: 171.

123   Ibid, Gabriel Cousens. "Iodine- The Universal & Holistic Super Mineral."

124   Kelly FC. *"Iodine in medicine and pharmacy since its discovery - 1811-1961."* Proc R Soc Med, 1961; 54:831-836.

125   Coindet JF. "Decouverte d'un nouveau remede contre le goitre." Ann Clin Phys, 1820; 15:49.

126   Gennaro AR. *Remington: The Science and Practice of Pharmacy. 19th edition.* Mack Publishing Co., 1995; 1267.

127   Pittman, *et al.* "Thyroidal radioiodine uptake." *NEJM*, 1969; 280:1431-1434.

128   Abraham, G.E. "The Safe and Effective Implementation of Orthoiodosupplementation In Medical Practice."

129   Abraham, G.E. "The Safe and Effective Implementation of Orthoiodosupplementation In Medical Practice."

130   Ibid., Abraham, Guy E., J. D. Flechas, and J. C. Hakala. "Optimum Levels of Iodine for Greatest Mental and Physical Health."

131   Abraham, G. E. "The Historical Background of the Iodine Project." *The Original Internist* 12.2 (2005): 57-66.

132   Corriher, Thomas. *The Truth About Table Salt and The Chemical Industry.* Rep. Health Wyze Media, 6 Dec. 2008. Web. <http://healthwyze.org/reports/115-the-truth-about-table-salt-and-the-chemical-industry>.

133   Wayne,E.J,. Koutras,D.A.. Alexander,W.D.. Clinical aspects of iodine metabolism, Philadelphia:F.A. Davis Company, 1964.

134   Braverman,L.E.. Iodine and the thyroid: 33 years of study. Thyroid 4 (3): 351-356, 1994.

135   Vagenakis,A.G.. Effects of iodides: clinical studies. Thyroid 1 (1): 59-63, 1990.

136   Paul,T., et al. The effect of small increases in dietary iodine on thyroid function in euthyroid subjects. Metabolism. 37:121-124, 1988.

137   Zaichick,V. Zaichick.S.. Normal human intrathyroidal iodine. Science of the Total Environment 206 (1):39-56, 1997.

138   Ibid. Flechas, Abraham G.E., J.D., and J. C. Hakala. "Iodine Sufficiency of the Whole Body."

139   Ghent, W. "Iodine Replacement in Fibrocystic Disease of the Breast." *Can. J.Surg.* 36 (1993): 453-60.

140   Brownstein, David. *Iodine: Why You Need It, Why You Can't Live without It*. West Bloomfield, MI: Medical Alternatives Press, 2009.

141   Botha, Leslie Carol. "PCOS Affects 10% of Women of Childbearing Age."*Holy Hormones Journal*. Holy Hormones Journal, 11 Dec. 2014. Web. <http://holyhormones.com/womens-health/polycystic-ovarian-syndrome/pcos-affects-10-of-women-of-childbearing-age/>.

142   Derry, David M. *Breast Cancer and Iodine*. Victoria, B.C.: Trafford, 2001.

143   *Thyrodine, Physiology of Iodine*, pp.1-5. *Thyroidinstitute.org*. Compiled by W. Robert Doenges.

144   Abraham, Guy E., MD, George D. Flechas, MD, and John C. Hakala, R.Ph. "IODINE: Orthoiodosupplementation: Iodine Sufficiency Of The Whole Human Body." *IODINE:*

Orthoiodosupplementation: Iodine Sufficiency Of The Whole Human Body. Optimox, n.d. Web. 17 Jan. 2016.

145 Ghandrakant, C. et al. "Breast Cancer Relationship to Thyroid Supplements for hypothyroidism." *JAMA*, 238:1124, 1976.

146 Smyth, P. "Thyroid Disease and Breast Cancer," *J. Endo. Int.*, 16:396-401, 1993

147 Eskin, B. et al. "Mammary Gland Dysplasia in Iodine Deficiency." *JAMA,* 200:115-119, 1967.

148 Eskin, B., Iodine Metabolism and Breast Cancer. Trans. New York, Acad. Of Sciences, 32:911-947, 1970.

149 Rossouw, Jacques E., MD, et al. "Risks and Benefits of Estrogen Plus Progestin in Healthy Postmenopausal Women: Principal Results From the Women's Health Initiative Randomized Controlled Trial." *JAMA: The Journal of the American Medical Association* 288, no. 3 (2002): 321-33. doi:10.1001/jama.288.3.321.

150 Rowan T. Chlebowski et al.; for the WHI Investigators. "Estrogen Plus Progestin and Breast Cancer Incidence and Mortality in Postmenopausal Women." *JAMA*, 2010; 304 (15): 1684-1692 DOI: 10.1001/jama.2010.1500.

151 Ghandrakant, C. et al. "Breast Cancer. Relationship to Thyroid Supplements for Hypothyroidism." *JAMA: The Journal of the American Medical Association* 236, no. 10 (1976): 1124-127. doi:10.1001/jama.236.10.1124.

152 Hollowell J. et al., "Iodine Nutrition in the United States. Trends and Public Health Implications: Iodine Excretion Data from National Health and Nutrition Examination Surveys I and III" (1971-1974 and 1988-1994) J. *Clinical Endocrinology and Metabolism*, 83:3401-3408, 1998.

153 Brownstein, David, MD. "Taking Thyroid Hormone Increases Breast Cancer Risk By 200% « Dr. Brownstein." Dr Brownstein RSS. http://blog.drbrownstein.com/taking-thyroid-hormone-increases-breast-cancer-risk-by-200/.

154 Silva, Veronica et al. "Effect of Cell Phone-like Electromagnetic Radiation on Primary Human Thyroid Cells." *International Journal of Radiation Biology* (2015): 1-9.

155 Sadetzki, S., A. Chetrit, A. Jarus-Hakak, E. Cardis, et al. "Cellular Phone Use and Risk of Benign and Malignant Parotid Gland Tumors—A Nationwide Case-Control Study." *American Journal of Epidemiology* 167.4 (2008): 457-67.

156 Cancer Care Ontario. Cancer Fact: Thyroid cancer driving the rise in cancers in young women. April 2013. Available at http://www.cancercare.on.ca/cancerfacts/.

157 Davies L, Welch HG. "Increasing incidence of thyroid cancer in the United States, 1973–2002." *JAMA.* 2006: 295:2164–7. [PubMed]

158 Hyeong Sik Ahn et al. Korea's Thyroid-Cancer "Epidemic" — Screening and Overdiagnosis. N Engl J Med 2014; 371:1765-1767 November 6, 2014. DOI: 10.1056/NEJMp1409841.

159 "Do We Know What Causes Thyroid Cancer?" *Do We Know What Causes Thyroid Cancer?* American Cancer Society, n.d. Web. 17 Jan. 2016.

160 Peterson, M. "Hyperthyroidism in Cats: What's Causing This Epidemic of Thyroid Disease and Can We Prevent It?" *J Feline Med Surg.* 14, no. 11 (November 2012): 804-18. doi:10.1177/1098612X12464462.

161 INTERNATIONAL COUNCIL FOR CONTROL OF

IODINE DEFICIENCY DISORDERS, May 2007 Newsletter, Volume 24 [Newsletter]

162 Hartoft-Nielsen, Marie-Louise, et al. "Do Thyroid Disrupting Chemicals Influence Foetal Development during Pregnancy?" *Journal of Thyroid Research* 2011 (2011): 1-14. Web. <http://www.ncbi.nlm.nih.gov/pmc/articles/PMC3170895/#B27>.

163 Li, Creswell, J Eastman, et al., "Are Australian children iodine deficient? Results of the Australian National Iodine Nutrition Study," *MJA* 2006; 184 (4): 165-169.

164 Travers CA, et al. "Iodine status in pregnant women and their newborns: are our babies at risk of iodine deficiency?" *Med J Aust*. 2006;184:617–620.

165 McElduff A et al. "Neonatal thyroid-stimulating hormone concentrations in northern Sydney: further indications of mild iodine deficiency?" *Med J Aust* 2002; 176: 317-320. <eMJA full text>

166 Li M, Ma G, Guttikonda K, et al. "Re-emergence of iodine deficiency in Australia." *Asia Pac J Clin Nutr* 2001; 10: 200-203. <PubMed>

167 Hynes KL et al. "Persistent iodine deficiency in a cohort of Tasmanian school children: associations with socio-economic status, geographical location and dietary factors." *Aust N Z J Public Health* 2004; 28: 476-481. <PubMed>

168 Guttikonda K, Travers C, Lewis P, Boyages S. "Iodine deficiency in urban school children: a cross-sectional analysis." *Med J Aust* 2003; 179: 346-348. <eMJA full text> <PubMed>

169 Parnell, Winsome. *NZ Food NZ Children: Key Results of the 2002 National Children's Nutrition Survey*. Wellington, N.Z.: Ministry of Health, 2003. *The 2002 National Children's Nutrition Survey*.

Ministry of Health, 2002. https://www.health.govt.nz/system/ files/documents/publications/nzfoodnzchildren.pdf

170   Delange F., Eur J Nucl Med Mol Imaging, *Iodine deficiency in Europe and its Consequences*: an update., 2002, Aug 29 Suppl 2:S404-16.

171   Kumar, S. "Indicators to Monitor Progress of National Iodine Deficiency Disorders Control Programme (NIDDCP) and Some Observations on Iodised Salt in West Bengal." *Indian J Public Health* 39.4 (1995): 141-7.

172   Tiwari, B. K., A. K. Kundu, and R. D. Bansai. "National Iodine Deficiency Disorders Control Programme in India." *Indian J Public Health* 39.4 (1995): 148-51.

173   Finley JW., Bogardus, G.M., Breast Cancer and Thyroid Disease Quart. Review Surg. Obstet. Gyn. 17:139-147, 1960.

174   Silva, C. M., and M. V. Souza. "Autoimmune Hypothyroidism Nonresponsive to High Doses of Levothyroxine and Severe Hypocalcemia." *Arg Bras Endocrinol Metabol* 49.4 (2005): 599-603.

175   Beld, Annewieke et al. "Thyroid Hormone Concentrations, Disease, Physical Function, and Mortality in Elderly Men." *The Journal of Clinical Endocrinology & Metabolism* 90.12 (2005): 6403-409.

176   Chan SY, Vasilopoulou E, Kilby MD. The role of the placenta in thyroid hormone delivery to the fetus.*Nature Clinical Practice Endocrinology and Metabolism.* 2009;5 (1):45–54.

177   Koopdonk-kool JM, De Vijlder JJM, Veenboer GJM, et al. "Type II and type III deiodinase activity in human placenta as a function of gestational age." *Journal of Clinical Endocrinology and Met abolism.*1996;81(6):2154–2158.

178 Bernal J , Nunez J . Thyroid hormones and brain development. *Eur J Endocrinol*1995;133:390–8.

179 Ahmed O.M. et al..Thyroid hormones states and brain development interactions. *Int J Dev Neurosci* 2008;26:147–209.

180 Haddow JE , Palomaki GE. et al. Maternal thyroid deficiency during pregnancy and subsequent neuropsychological development of the child.*N Engl J Med*1999;**341**:549–55.

181 Pop VJ , Kuijpens JL et al. Low maternal free thyroxine concentrations during early pregnancy are associated with impaired psychomotor development in infancy.*Clin Endocrinol (Oxf)*1999;**50**:149–55.

182 Vermiglio, F. et al. "Attention Deficit and Hyperactivity Disorders in the Offspring of Mothers Exposed to Mild-Moderate Iodine Deficiency: A Possible Novel Iodine Deficiency Disorder in Developed Countries." *The Journal of Clinical Endocrinology & Metabolism* 89.12 (2004): 6054-060.

183 Journal Thyroid (Vol. 19, N9, 2009, published ahead of print 8.13.09).

184 *Centers for Disease Control and Prevention.* Centers for Disease Control and Prevention, 10 Sept. 2015.

185 "Hypothyroidism in Infants and Children / Thyroid Disease Information Source - Articles/FAQs." *Hypothyroidism in Infants and Children / Thyroid Disease Information Source - Articles/FAQs.*

186 Shomon, Mary J. *Living Well with Hypothyroidism: What Your Doctor Doesn't Tell You ... That You Need to Know.* New York: HarperResource, 2005.

187 de Onis M., Monteiro C., Akré J., Clugston G. The worldwide magnitude of protein-energy malnutrition: an overview from

the WHO global database on child growth. WHO Bull. 1993; 71:703-712.

188   Cuttler, L., Singh, J., Silvers, J.B., O'Connor, K. & Neuhauser, D. (1994). "Growth hormone as a treatment of short stature in children: the scope of the issue." *International Society of Technology Assessment in Health Care Meeting.* Abstract No. 163.

189   Beek, Nina Van, Enikő Bodó, et al. "Thyroid Hormones Directly Alter Human Hair Follicle Functions: Anagen Prolongation and Stimulation of Both Hair Matrix Keratinocyte Proliferation and Hair Pigmentation." *The Journal of Clinical Endocrinology & Metabolism* 93.11 (2008): 4381-388.

190   Flechas, George. "Iodine Insufficiency FAQ." *Flechas Family Practice.* N.p., n.d.

191   Khurana KK, Labrador E, Izquierdo R, et al. "The role of fine-needle aspiration biopsy in the management of thyroid nodules in children, adolescents, and young adults: a multi-institutional study." *Thyroid.* Apr 1999;9(4):383-6. [Medline].

192   Albright JT, Topham AK, Reilly JS. "Pediatric head and neck malignancies: US incidence and trends over 2 decades." *Arch Otolaryngol Head Neck Surg.* Jun 2002;128(6):655-9. [Medline].

193   Miccoli P. et al. Papillary thyroid cancer: pathological parameters as prognostic factors in different classes of age. *Otolaryngol Head Neck Surg.* Feb 2008;138(2):200-3. [Medline].

194   Silverman SH, Nussbaum M, Rausen AR. "Thyroid nodules in children: a ten year experience at one institution." *Mt Sinai J Med.* Sep-Oct 1979;46(5):460-3. [Medline].

195   Attie JA. Carcinoma of the thyroid in children and adolescents. In: F Lifshitz. *Pediatric Endocrinology.* 3. New York: Marcel Dekker; 1996:423–432.

196   Schneider K. Sonographic imaging of the thyroid in children. *Prog Pediatr Surg.* 1991;26:1-14. [Medline].

197   Sherman NH, Rosenberg HK, Heyman S, et al. "Ultrasound evaluation of neck masses in children." *J Ultrasound Med.* Mar 1985;4(3):127-34. [Medline].

198   Joppich I, Roher HD, Hecker WC, et al. "Thyroid carcinoma in childhood." *Prog Pediatr Surg.* 1983;16:23-8. [Medline].

199   Garcia CJ, Daneman A, Thorner P, et al. Sonography of multinodular thyroid gland in children and adolescents. *Am J Dis Child.* Jul 1992;146(7):811-6. [Medline].

200   Bethell, CD, Kogan, MD, et al. 2011. A national and state profile of leading health problems and health care quality for US children: key insurance disparities and across-state variations. Acad Pediatr. May-June; 11(3 Suppl): S22-33.

201   Summary Health Statistics for U.S. Children: National Health Interview Survey, 2012, table 2. http://www.cdc.gov/nchs/data/series/sr_10/sr10_258.pdf

202   Devereux G. 2006. The increase in the prevalence of asthma and allergy: food for thought. Nat Rev Immunol. Nov; 6(11):869-74.

203   Pastor, P. N., & Reuben, C. A. (2008). Diagnosed attention deficit hyperactivity disorder and learning disability: United States, 2004-2006. *Vital and Health Statistics, 10.* Retrieved June 26, 2012, from http://www.cdc.gov/nchs/data/series/sr_10/Sr10_237.pdf

204   Narayan, K. M. Venkat. "Lifetime Risk for Diabetes Mellitus in the United States." *Jama* 290.14 (2003): 1884.

205   Zablotsky, B., L. I. Black, M. J. Maenner, L. A. Schieve, and S. J. Blumberg, *Estimated Prevalence of Autism and Other*

Developmental Disabilities Following Questionnaire Changes in the 2014 National Health Interview Survey. Rep. no. 87. CDC National Health Statistics Reports, 13 Nov. 2015. Web

206   Williams KV, Nayak S, Becker D, et al. *"Fifty years of experience with propylthiouracil-associated hepatotoxicity: What have we learned?" J Clin Endocr & Metab,* 1997; 82:1727-1733.

207   Cooper DS. *"Treatment of Thyrotoxicosis." In:* Werner & Ingbar's The Thyroid. Braverman LE and Utiger RD, editors. Lippincott Williams & Wilkins, 2000; 691-715.

208   Alexander, W. D., and Sheenah K. Bisset. "The Correlation Of Thyroid Function With The Rate Of Oxygen Uptake Of Human Leucocytes." *Quarterly Journal of Experimental Physiology and Cognate Medical Sciences,* vol. 46, no. 1, 1961, pp. 46–49., doi:10.1113/expphysiol.1961.sp001514.

209   Broberg K. et al. Lithium in drinking water and thyroid function. *Environmental Health Perspectives.* 2011;119(6):827–830. [PMC free article] [PubMed]

210   Brownstein, David. "Iodine: Why You Need It, Why You Can't Live without It." West Bloomfield, MI: Medical Alternatives, 2009.

211   Hirzy, J. William et al. "Comparison of hydrofluorosilicic acid and pharmaceutical sodium fluoride as fluoridating agents—A cost–benefit analysis." *Environmental Science & Policy* 29 (May 2013): 81-86. doi:10.1016/j.envsci.2013.01.007.

212   Peckham, S., D. Lowery, and S. Spencer. "Are Fluoride Levels in Drinking Water Associated with Hypothyroidism Prevalence in England? A Large Observational Study of GP Practice Data and Fluoride Levels in Drinking Water." *Journal of Epidemiology & Community Health* 69.7 (2015): 619-24.

213   Young, Saundra. "Government Recommends Lowering Fluoride Levels in U.S. Drinking Water." *CNN.* Cable News Network, 07 Jan. 2011.

214   Chandu, Gn et al. "Prevalence and Severity of Dental Fluorosis among 13 to 15-year-old School Children of an Area Known for Endemic Fluorosis: Nalgonda District of Andhra Pradesh." *J Indian Soc Pedod Prev Dent Journal of Indian Society of Pedodontics and Preventive Dentistry* 27.4 (2009): 190. Web. <http://fluoride-alert.org/wp-content/uploads/sudhir-2009.pdf>.

215   Shivaprakash, Pk et al. "Relation between Dental Fluorosis and Intelligence Quotient in School Children of Bagalkot District." *J Indian Soc Pedod Prev Dent Journal of Indian Society of Pedodontics and Preventive Dentistry* 29.2 (2011): 117.

216   Dr. Philippe Grandjean, MD, Philip J. Landrigan, MD. "Neurobehavioural effects of developmental toxicity." The Lancet Neurology, Volume 13, Issue 3, Pages 330-338, March 2014. doi: 10.1016/S1474-4422(13)70278-3.

217   Martín-Pardillos, Ana, Cecilia Sosa, Ángel Millán, and Víctor Sorribas. "Effect of Water Fluoridation on the Development of Medial Vascular Calcification in Uremic Rats." *Toxicology* 318 (2014): 40-50. <http://www.ncbi.nlm.nih.gov/pubmed/24561004>.

218   Sayed, A. J. "Mania and Bromism: A Case Report and a Look to the Future." *American Journal of Psychiatry AJP* 133.2 (1976): 228-29.

219   Malenchenko AF, Demidchik EP, and Tadeush VN. "The content and distribution of iodine, chlorine and bromide in the normal and pathologically changed thyroid tissue." Med Radiol, 1984; 29:19-22.

220   Horowitz, B. Zane. "Bromism from Excessive Cola Consumption." *Journal of Toxicology: Clinical Toxicology* 35.3 (1997): 315-20.

221   Stapleton, Heather M. et al. "Identification of Flame Retardants in Polyurethane Foam Collected from Baby Products." *Environmental Science & Technology*, vol. 45, no. 12, 15 June 2011, pp. 5323–5331., doi:10.1021/es2007462.

222   Golomb, Beatrice Alexandra. *A Review of the Scientific Literature As It Pertains To Gulf War Illness*. Vol. 2. N.p.: RAND, 1999. *Chapter Ten: Bromism*. RAND. Web. 30 Jan. 2016. <http://www.gulflink.osd.mil/library/randrep/pb_paper/mr1018.2.chap10.html>.

223   Levin, Max. "Transitory Schizophrenias Produced By Bromide Intoxication." *American Journal of Psychiatry AJP* 103.2 (1946): 229-37.

224   Barrett, Julia R. "Thimerosal and Animal Brains: New Data for Assessing Human Ethylmercury Risk." *Environmental Health Perspectives*, vol. 113, no. 8, Jan. 2005, pp. A543–544., doi:10.1289/ehp.113-a543.

225   Menomune Package Insert. (2013, April). Retrieved from https://www.vaccineshoppe.com/image.cfm?doc_id=10447&image_type=product_pdf

226   Dórea, José G. "Low-dose Thimerosal in pediatric vaccines: Adverse effects in perspective." *Environmental Research*152 (January 2017): 280-93. doi:10.1016/j.envres.2016.10.028.

227   Aschner,, M., and S. J. Walker. "The neuropathogenesis of mercury toxicity." *Mol Psychiatry.*7, no. 2 (December 31, 2001): S40-1. http://www.nature.com/mp/journal/v7/n2s/pdf/4001176a.pdf.

228   Dórea, José. "Exposure to Mercury and Aluminum in Early

Life: Developmental Vulnerability as a Modifying Factor in Neurologic and Immunologic Effects." *International Journal of Environmental Research and Public Health*12, no. 2 (January 23, 2015): 1295-313. doi:10.3390/ijerph120201295.

229   Waly, M , H. et al. "Activation of methionine synthase by insulin-like growth factor-1 and dopamine: a target for neurodevelopmental toxins and thimerosal." *Molecular Psychiatry*, 2004, 1-13. http://progressiveconvergence.com/Activation%20of%20Methionine%20Synthase.pdf.

230   Barrett, J. R. (2005). Thimerosal and Animal Brains: New Data for Assessing Human Ethylmercury Risk. *Environ Health Perspect.,113*(8), A543-A544. Retrieved from https://www.ncbi.nlm.nih.gov/pmc/articles/PMC1280369/.

231   Blaylock, Russell, MD. "How Vaccines Can Damage Your Brain." Editorial. *VRAN Newsletter*, Spring 2008. http://www.whale.to/b/blaylock.html.

232   Havarinasab S et al. "Immunosuppressive and autoimmune effects of thimerosal in mice." *Toxicol Appl Pharmacol* 2005; 204: 109-121. https://www.researchgate.net/publication/7926842_Immunosuppressive_and_autoimmune_effects_of_thimerosal_in_mice

233   Heckenlively, Kent, Esq. "MERCURY, TESTOSTERONE AND AUTISM - A REALLY BIG IDEA!" Age Of Autism. April 21, 2008. http://www.ageofautism.com/2008/04/mercury-testost.html.

234   Miller, Neil Z. "Combining Childhood Vaccines at One Visit Is Not Safe." *Journal of American Physicians and Surgeons* 21.2 (2016): 47-49. Web. <http://www.rescuepost.com/files/n-miller-vaccines-article.pdf>.

235   Ma, Bo, Li-Fang He et al. "Characteristics and Viral Propagation Properties of a New Human Diploid Cell Line, Walvax-2, and Its Suitability as a Candidate Cell Substrate for Vaccine Production." *Human Vaccines & Immunotherapeutics* 11.4 (2015): 998-1009.

236   Theresa, A. Deisher, et al. "English." *J. Public Health Epidemiol. Journal of Public Health and Epidemiology* 6.9 (2014): 271-86.

237   Horner, L. M., Poulter, M. D., Brenton, J., & Turner, R. B. (2015). Acute Flaccid Paralysis Associated with Novel Enterovirus C105. *Emerging Infectious Diseases*, 21(10), 1858-1860. https://dx.doi.org/10.3201/eid2110.150759.

238   Cowling, B, J., Fang, V. J., Nishiura, H., Chan, K. H., Ng, S., Ip, D. K. M., Chiu, S. S., Leung, G. M., & Peiris, J. S. M. (2012, June 15). Increased Risk of Noninfluenza Respiratory Virus Infections Associated With Receipt of Inactivated Influenza Vaccine, *Clinical Infectious Diseases*, 54(12), 1778–1783. https://doi.org/10.1093/cid/cis307.

239   Read, A. F., Baigent, S. J., Powers, C., Kgosana, L.B., Blackwell, L., Smith, L.P., Kennedy, D.A., Walkden-Brown, S.W., & Nair, V. N. (2015, July 27). Imperfect Vaccination Can Enhance the Transmission of Highly Virulent Pathogens. *PLOS Biology* 13(7). https://doi.org/10.1371/journal.pbio.1002198.

240   Benjamin M. Althouse and Samuel V. Scarpino. *"Asymptomatic transmission and the resurgence of Bordetella pertussis."* BMC *Medicine*, 2015; 13 (1) DOI: 10.1186/s12916-015-0382-8

241   Dunn, Glynis, and Dimitra Klapsa. "Twenty-Eight Years of Poliovirus Replication in an Immunodeficient Individual: Impact on the Global Polio Eradication Initiative." *PLoS Pathog PLOS Pathogens* 11.8 (2015).

242   Giangaspero, M. et al. (2001). "Genotypes of pestivirus RNA

detected in live virus vaccines for human use." *J Vet Med Sci.*, 67(7), 623-33. Retrieved from https://www.ncbi.nlm.nih.gov/pubmed/11503899.

243   Gibson, Daniel G. et al. "Creation of a Bacterial Cell Controlled by a Chemically Synthesized Genome." *Science*329, no. 5987, (July 2, 2010): 52-56. doi:10.1126/science.1190719.

244   Rappoport, Jon. "New Vaccines Will Permanently Alter Human DNA." New Vaccines Will Permanently Alter Human DNA. January 01, 1970. http://humansarefree.com/2016/05/new-vaccines-will-permanently-alter.html.

245   Krawitz, Christian et al. "Inhibitory activity of a standardized elderberry liquid extract against clinically-Relevant human respiratory bacterial pathogens and influenza A and B viruses." *BMC Complementary and Alternative Medicine*, vol. 11, no. 1, 2011, doi:10.1186/1472-6882-11-16.

246   Lehtoranta, L. "Probiotics in respiratory virus infections." *Eur J Clin Microbiol Infect Dis.* , vol. 33, no. 8, Aug. 2014, pp. 1289–1302., doi:10.1007/s10096-014-2086-y.

247   Date K, Ohno K. et al. Endocrine-disrupting effects of styrene oligomers that migrated from polystyrene containers into food. *Food and Chemical Toxicology.* 2002;40(1):65–75. [PubMed]

248   Divi RL, Chang HC, Doerge DR. "Anti-thyroid isoflavones from soybean. Isolation, characterization, and mechanisms of action." *Biochemical Pharmacology.* 1997;54(10):1087–1096. [PubMed]

249   Ardies, C.m., and C. Dees. "Xenoestrogens Significantly Enhance Risk for Breast Cancer during Growth and Adolescence." *Medical Hypotheses* 50.6 (1998): 457-64. Web. June 1998. <http://www.ncbi.nlm.nih.gov/pubmed/9710315>.

250 C. E. Counsell, A. Taha, and W. S. J. Ruddell, "Coeliac disease and autoimmune thyroid disease," Gut, vol. 35, no. 6, pp. 844–846, 1994.

251 A. Ventura et al. "Gluten-dependent diabetes-related and thyroid-related autoantibodies in patients with celiac disease," Journal of Pediatrics, vol. 137, no. 2, pp. 263–265, 2000.

252 D. Larizza et al., "Celiac disease in children with autoimmune thyroid disease," Journal of Pediatrics, vol. 139, no. 5, pp. 738–740, 2001.

253 Pynnonen PA, Isometsa ET, Verkasalo MA, Kahkonen SA, Sipila I, Savilahti E, Aalberg VA. Gluten-free diet may alleviate depressive and behavioural symptoms in adolescents with coeliac disease: a prospective follow-up case-series study. BMC Psychiatry. 2005;5:14.

254 Pals, Maria Van Der et al. "Prevalence of Thyroid Autoimmunity in Children with Celiac Disease Compared to Healthy 12-Year Olds." Autoimmune Diseases 2014 (2014): 1-6.

255 Sategna-Guidetti, C., and U. Volta. "Prevalence of Thyroid Disorders in Untreated Adult Celiac Disease Patients and Effect of Gluten Withdrawal: An Italian Multicenter Study." Am J Gastroenterol. 96.3 (2001): 751-7.

256 A. Ventura, E. Neri, C. et al. "Gluten-dependent diabetes-related and thyroid-related autoantibodies in patients with celiac disease," Journal of Pediatrics, vol. 137, no. 2, pp. 263–265, 2000.

257 D. Larizza et al., "Celiac disease in children with autoimmune thyroid disease," Journal of Pediatrics, vol. 139, no. 5, pp. 738–740, 2001.

258 Silva, C. M., and M. V. Souza. "[Autoimmune Hypothyroidism Nonresponsive to High Doses of Levothyroxine and Severe

Hypocalcemia]." *Arq Bras Endocrinol Metabol.* 49.4 (2005): 599-603.

259 Spadaccino, Aglaura Cinzia et al. "Celiac Disease in North Italian Patients with Autoimmune Thyroid Diseases." *Autoimmunity* 41.1 (2008): 116-21.

260 Luorio, L., Mercuri V. et al. "Prevalence of Celiac Disease in Patients with Autoimmune Thyroiditis." *Minerva Endocrinol.* 32.4 (2007): 239-43.

261 Adams, Scott. "Early Diagnosis of Gluten Sensitivity: Before the Villi are Gone by, By Kenneth Fine, M.D." Early Diagnosis of Gluten Sensitivity: Before the Villi are Gone by By Kenneth Fine, M.D. - Celiac.com. March 03, 2004. https://www.celiac.com/articles/759/1/Early-Diagnosis-of-Gluten-Sensitivity-Before-the-Villi-are-Gone-by-By-Kenneth-Fine-MD/Page1.html.

262 Amasheh, Maren, et al., "TNF⊠-induced and berberine-antago-nized tight junction barrier impairment via tyrosine kinase, Akt and NF⊠B signaling." *Journal of Cell Science* 123.23 (2010):4145-4155. doi:jcs.biologists.org/content/123/23/4145.long.

263 Greco, Luigi et al. "Safety for Patients With Celiac Disease of Baked Goods Made of Wheat Flour Hydrolyzed During Food Processing." Clinical Gastroenterology and Hepatology 9, no. 1 (2011): 24-29. doi:10.1016/j.cgh.2010.09.025.

264 Samsel, Anthony, and Stephanie Seneff. "Glyphosate's Suppression of Cytochrome P450 Enzymes and Amino Acid Biosynthesis by the Gut Microbiome: Pathways to Modern Diseases." Entropy 15, no. 4 (2013): 1416-463. doi:10.3390/e15041416.

265 "The Health Dangers of Roundup (glyphosate) Herbicide. Jeffrey Smith & Stephanie Seneff." Interview by Jeffrey Smith and

Stephanie Seneff. *The Institute for Responsible Technology*. N.p., 10 May 2013.

266   Bressan, Paola, and Peter Kramer. "Bread and Other Edible Agents of Mental Disease." *Frontiers in Human Neuroscience Front. Hum. Neurosci.* 10 (2016): n. pag. Web. <http://www.ncbi. nlm.nih.gov/pmc/articles/PMC4809873/>.

267   Sategna-Guidetti, C., and U. Volta. "Prevalence of Thyroid Disorders in Untreated Adult Celiac Disease Patients and Effect of Gluten Withdrawal: An Italian Multicenter Study." *Am J Gastroenterol.* 96, no. 3 (March 2001): 751-7.

268   YouTube. August 31, 2016. https://www.youtube.com/embed/ k33iFXHlOnY.

269   Honeycutt, Zen. "Glyphosate in Childhood Vaccines." Moms Across America. September 6, 2016. http://www.momsacrossa- merica.com/glyphosate_in_childhood_vaccines.

270   Zen Honeycutt, Henry Rowlands, Lori Grace. "Glyphosate Testing Full Report: Findings in American Mothers' Breast Milk, Urine and Water," Moms Across America. April 7, 2015 http://www.momsacrossamerica.com/glyphosate_testing_results.

271   Wartofsky L. *"Has the use of antithyroid drugs for Graves' disease become obsolete ?"* Thyroid, 1993; 3:335-344.

272   "Research on Brain and Biological Effects of Cell-Phones." *Research on Brain and Biological Effects of Cell-Phones.* N.p., n.d. Web. 06 July 2016. <http://dynamics.org/Altenberg/MED/ CELL_PHONES/>.

273   Sadetzki, S., A. Chetrit, et al. "Cellular Phone Use and Risk of Benign and Malignant Parotid Gland Tumors—A Nationwide Case-Control Study." *American Journal of Epidemiology*167.4

(2008): 457-67. Web. 08 Oct. 2007. <http://aje.oxfordjournals. org/content/167/4/457>.

274   Hardell, L. et al. "Long-term Use of Cellular Phones and Brain Tumours: Increased Risk Associated with Use for =10 Years." *Occupational and Environmental Medicine*64.9 (2007): 626-32. Web. 28 Mar. 2007.

275   Ron E. "Thyroid cancer incidence among people living in areas contaminated by radiation from the Chernobyl accident." *Health Phys.* Nov 2007;93(5):502-11. [Medline].

276   Mary Felber et al. Amplification of the c-myc Oncogene in Radiation-Induced Rat Skin Tumors as a Function of Linear Energy Transfer and Dose, *Radiation Research*, Vol. 131, No. 3 (Sep., 1992), pp. 297-301 (article consists of 5 pages), Published by: Radiation Research Society

277   Festen C, et al. "Follicular adenoma of the thyroid gland in children." *Eur J Pediatr Surg.* Oct 1995;5(5):262-4. [Medline].

278   Vane, D., King, D.R., & Boles Jr., E.T. (December 1984). Secondary thyroid neoplasms in pediatric cancer patients: increased risk with improved survival. Journal of Pediatric Surgery, 19(6), 855-60. Retrieved from https://www.ncbi.nlm. nih.gov/pubmed/6097662.

279   Sklar C, Whitton J. et al. "Abnormalities of the thyroid in survivors of Hodgkin's disease: data from the Childhood Cancer Survivor Study." *J Clin Endocrinol Metab.* Sep 2000;85(9):3227-32. [Medline].

280   "U.S. Breast Cancer Statistics | Breastcancer.org." *Breastcancer. org.* N.p., n.d. Web. http://www.breastcancer.org/symptoms/ understand_bc/statistics.

281   Henderson, L. M., R. A. et al. "Increased Risk of Developing Breast Cancer after a False-Positive Screening Mammogram." *Cancer Epidemiology Biomarkers & Prevention* 24.12 (2015): 1882-889. Web. 2 Dec. 2015. <http://cebp.aacrjournals.org/content/early/2015/11/09/1055-9965.EPI-15-0623.abstract>.

282   Gøtzsche, P. C., and K. Jorgenson. "Cochrane." *Screening for Breast Cancer with Mammography | Cochrane.* Cochrane, 4 June 2013. Web. <http://www.cochrane.org/CD001877/BREASTCA_screening-for-breast-cancer-with-mammography>.

283   Begley, Sharon. "Could This Be The End Of Cancer?" *Newsweek.* N.p., 14 Dec. 2011. Web. <http://www.newsweek.com/could-be-end-cancer-65869>.

284   Moscicki, Anna-Barbara et al. "Regression of Low-grade Squamous Intra-epithelial Lesions in Young Women." *The Lancet* 364.9446 (2004): 1678-683. Web. <http://www.thelancet.com/journals/lancet/article/PIIS0140-6736%2804%2917354-6/fulltext#article_upsell>.

285   Frenkel, M. et al. "Cytotoxic effects of ultra-Diluted remedies on breast cancer cells." *International Journal of Oncology*, vol. 36, no. 2, 2009, doi:10.3892/ijo_00000512.

286   Suberblelle, Elsa et al. "DNA Repair Factor BRCA1 Depletion Occurs in Alzheimer Brains and Impairs Cognitive Function in Mice." *Nature Communications* 6.8897, 2015.

287   Murphy, Brendan D. "SCIENCE MEETS SPIRITUALITY." *Science Meets Spirituality*(n.d.): n. pag. *Http://www.bibliotecapleyades.net/.* Web. p.10 <http://www.bibliotecapleyades.net/archivos_pdf/science-meets-spirituality.pdf>.

288   Cossetti, Cristina et al. "Soma-to-Germline Transmission of

RNA in Mice Xenografted with Human Tumour Cells: Possible Transport by Exosomes." *PLoS ONE* 9.7. 2014.

289   Fosar, Grazyna, and Franz Bludorf. "You Are Being Redirected..." *You Are Being Redirected...* Zengardener.com, n.d. Web. 17 Jan. 2016.

290   Abate, Tom. "News Stories About Tinkering With DNA Miss the Big Picture / Glowing Rabbit Shows We're Creeping toward Redesigning Human Life." *SFGate.* San Francisco Gate, 25 Sept. 2000. Web. <http://www.sfgate.com/business/article/News-Stories-About-Tinkering-With-DNA-Miss-the-3303065.php>.

291   Eschowsky, Myron. "Question on Soul Separation." *Question on Soul Separation*, 2 Feb. 2017.

292   Eshowsky, Myron. *Peace with Cancer: Shamanism as a Spiritual Approach to Healing.* Shoshana Publications, 2009.

293   Samuels, Mike, and Mary Rockwood. Lane. *Shaman Wisdom, Shaman Healing: Deepen Your Ability to Heal with Visionary and Spiritual Tools and Practices.* Hoboken, NJ: John Wiley & Sons, 2003. Print.

294   Clayton, Paul, PhD, and Judith Rowbotam. "Forget Paleo, Go Mid-Victorian: It's the Healthiest Diet You've Never Heard of." *Spectator Health.* The Spectator, 12 Nov. 2015.

295   Hess, Evelyn V. "Environmental Chemicals and Autoimmune Disease: Cause and Effect." *Toxicology* 181-182, 2002: 65-70.

296   Taubes, Gary. *Good Calories, Bad Calories: Fats, Carbs, and the Controversial Science of Diet and Health.* New York: Anchor, 2008. Print.

297   Hertog MGL, Feskens EJM, Hollman PCH, Katan MB, Kromhout D. Dietary antioxidantflavonoids and risk of coronary

heart disease. The Zutphen Elderly Study. <u>Lancet 1993;342:1007-1012.</u> Impact factor = 39.1; Citations: 2579

298   Berg, Jeremy M. "Important Derivatives of Cholesterol Include Bile Salts and Steroid Hormones." *NCBI*. U.S. National Library of Medicine, 2002. Web. 17 Aug. 2016. <http://www.ncbi.nlm.nih.gov/books/NBK22339/>.

299   Mozaffarian, Dariush et al. "Dietary Fats, Carbohydrate, and Progression of Coronary Atherosclerosis in Postmenopausal Women." *Am J Clin Nutr*. 80.5 (2004): 1175-84. Web. <http://www.ncbi.nlm.nih.gov/pmc/articles/PMC1270002/>.

300   Mielke, M. M., P. et al.. "High Total Cholesterol Levels in Late Life Associated with a Reduced Risk of Dementia." *Neurology* 64.10 (2005): 1689-695. Web. <http://www.ncbi.nlm.nih.gov/pubmed/15911792>.

301   Hamazaki, T. et al. "Towards a Paradigm Shift in Cholesterol Treatment." *Ann Nutr Metab.*, vol. 66, no. 4, 2015, pp. 1–116., doi:10.1159/isbn.978-3-318-05481-1.

302   Okuyama, Harumi et al. "Statins Stimulate Atherosclerosis and Heart Failure: Pharmacological Mechanisms." *Expert Review of Clinical Pharmacology* 8.2 (2015): 189-99. Web. <http://www.ncbi.nlm.nih.gov/pubmed/25655639/>.

303   Bliss, Michael (professor Of History, University Of Toronto. *William Osler - a Life in Medicine.* Oxford University Press Inc, 2007.

304   Realmilk.com. "The Milk Cure: Real Milk Cures Many Diseases." *A Campaign for Real Milk*, 4 Feb. 2014, www.realmilk.com/health/milk-cure/.

305   "Consumers - The Dangers of Raw Milk: Unpasteurized Milk Can Pose a Serious Health Risk." *U S Food and Drug*

Administration Home Page, Center for Food Safety and Applied Nutrition, 15 Nov. 2017.

306 Tacket CO, Narain JP, Sattin R, Lofgren JP, Konigsberg C Jr, Rendtorff RC, et al. A multistate outbreak of infections caused by *Yersinia enterocolitica* transmitted by pasteurized milk. JAMA. 1984;251:483–6 10.1001/jama.251.4.483.

307 Ackers ML, Schoenfeld S, Markman J, Smith MG, Nicholson MA, DeWitt W, et al. An outbreak of *Yersinia enterocolitica* O:8 infections associated with pasteurized milk. J Infect Dis. 2000;181:1834–7 10.1086/315436.

308 Black RE, Jackson RJ, Tsai T, Medvesky M, Shayegani M, Feeley J, et al. Epidemic *Yersinia enterocolitica* infection due to contaminated chocolate milk. N Engl J Med. 1978;298:76–9 10.1056/NEJM197801122980204.

309 Salmonella Gastroenteritis Associated with Milk — Arizona. (1979). Morbidity and Mortality Weekly Report, 28(10), 117-120. Retrieved from http://www.jstor.org/stable/23295541.

310 Fleming DW et al. "Pasteurized milk as a vehicle of infection in an outbreak of listeriosis." *N Engl J Med.* 1985;312:404–7 10.1056/NEJM198502143120704.

311 Birkhead G. et al., "A multiple-strain outbreak of Campylobacter enteritis due to consumption of inadequately pasteurized milk." *J Infect Dis.* 1988;157:1095–7.

312 Lindqvist, P.G., Epstein, E., Nielsen, K., Landin-Olsson, M., Ingvar, C. & Olsson, H. (2016). "Avoidance of sun exposure as a risk factor for major causes of death: a competing risk analysis of the Melanoma in Southern Sweden cohort." Journal of Internal Medicine, 280(4), 375-87. doi:10.1111/joim.12496.

313   Dextreit, Raymond, and Michel Abehsera. *Our Earth, Our Cure.* Swan House Pub. Co., 1974.

314   Villoldo, A. (2001) *Shaman, healer, sage: how to heal yourself and others with the energy medicine of the Americas.* Bantam.

315   Hutchens, Alma R. *Handbook of Native American Herbs.* Shambhala, 1992.

316   Brandt, Barbara Allys. "Homeopathy, Element-Remedies, and the Atomic Messages: How a client's healing experience opened up a new field of knowledge." *Atomic Messages Foundation*, August 29, 2015. http://www.elementmessages.com/pdfs/2015,%20 August%2029—article_homeopathy_elements.pdf.

317   Brandt, Barbara Allys. "Science and Spirituality in the Elements of the Periodic Table: The Elements' Deeper Meanings for our Lives (Publication)." *Atomic Messages Foundation,* June 3, 2016. http://www.elementmessages.com/pdfs/2016-june—3-science-spiirituality.pdf

318   ibid. Barbara A. Brandt, *Science and Spirituality in the Elements of the Periodic Table: The Elements' Deeper Meanings for our Lives.*

319   Barona, J L. "The body republic: social order and human body in Renaissance medical thought." *Hist Philos Life Sci.*, vol. 15, no. 2, 1993, pp. 165–80., www.ncbi.nlm.nih.gov/pubmed/8153261.

320   Grant, Evan. "Making Sound Visible through Cymatics." *Evan Grant:.* Tedx,Web. <http://www.ted.com/talks/evan_grant_cymatics?language=en#t-125957>.

321   "Water: Enough, More, or Less." *JAMA* 86 (June 19, 1926). doi:doi:10.1001/jama.1926.0267051003401

322   *Ethan A. Perets and Elsa C. Y. Yan, "The H2O Helix: The Chiral*

Water Superstructure Surrounding DNA." ACS Central Science *2017* 3 *(7)*, *683-685.* DOI: *10.1021/acscentsci.7b00229*

323 Cai, Na, Simon Chang et al. "Molecular Signatures of Major Depression." *Current Biology* 25, no. 9 (2015): 1146-156. doi:10.1016/j.cub.2015.03.008.

324 McCraty, R., PhD et al. "Modulation of DNA Conformation by Heart-Focused Intention ." *Institute of HeartMath.* http://www. aipro.info/drive/File/224.pdf.

325 *Water, the Great Mystery.* Directed by Saida Medvedeva. USA and Canada: Intention Media Inc.

326 Emoto, Masaru. *The Hidden Messages in Water.* Hillsboro: Beyond words Pub., 2004.

327 Emoto, Marasu, and Konstantin Korotkov, Ph.D. *Baikal Water Ceremony, August 3, 2008.* Report. July 9, 2012. http://korotkov. org/baikal-water-ceremony/#more-756.

328 Collings, P.J. *Liquid Crystals, Nature's Delicate Phase of Matter,* Princeton University Press, Princeton, 1990.

329 Blinov, L.M. *Electro-optical and Magneto-optical Principles of Liquid Crystals,* John Wiley and Sons, London, 1983.

330 Ho, Mae-Wan et al. "Organisms as Polyphasic Liquid Crystals." *Bioelectrochemistry and Bioenergetics* 41 (1996): 81-91. *Institute of Science in Society ISIS.* Web. <http://www.i-sis.org.uk/polypha. php>.

331 Kolesnikov, Alexander I. et al. "Quantum Tunneling of Water in Beryl: A New State of the Water Molecule." *Phys. Rev. Lett. Physical Review Letters* 116.16 (2016): n. pag. *Phys. Rev. Lett.* American Physical Society, 22 Apr. 2016. Web. <http://journals. aps.org/prl/abstract/10.1103/PhysRevLett.116.167802>.

332   Pollack, Gerald H. *The Fourth Phase of Water: Beyond Solid, Liquid, and Vapor.* Seattle, WA: Ebner & Sons, 2013. Print.

333   Aratani S, Fujita H. et al. "Murine hypothalamic destruction with vascular cell apoptosis subsequent to combined administration of human papilloma virus vaccine and pertussis toxin." *Sci Rep.* 2016 Nov 11;6:36943. doi: 10.1038/srep36943. https://www.ncbi.nlm.nih.gov/pmc/articles/PMC5105142/

334   Clements-Cortes, et al. "Short-Term Effects of Rhythmic Sensory Stimulation in Alzheimer's Disease: An Exploratory Pilot Study." *Journal of Alzheimer's Disease JAD* 52.2 (2016): 651-60. *J Alzheimers Dis.* PubMed, 25 Mar. 2016. Web. <10.3233/JAD-160081>.

335   Dextreit, Raymond, and Michel Abehsera. *Our Earth, Our Cure.* Brooklyn: Swan House Pub., 1974. Print.

336   Sharma, Ashok Kumar, Indraneel Basu, and Siddarth Singh. "Efficacy and Safety of Ashwagandha Root Extract in Subclinical Hypothyroid Patients: A Double-Blind, Randomized Placebo-Controlled Trial." *The Journal of Alternative and Complementary Medicine*, 2017. doi:10.1089/acm.2017.0183.

337   Chen, Chunqiu, et al. "Effects of berberine in the gastrointestinal tract—A review of actions and therapeutic implications." *The American Journal of Chinese Medicine* 42.05 (2014): 1053-1070. Effects of berberine in the gastrointestinal tract Chen Chunqiu 2014.

338   Peng WH1 et al. "Berberine produces antidepressant-like effects in the forced swim test and in the tail suspension test in mice." *Life Sci.* 2007 Aug 23;81(11):933-8. Epub 2007 Aug 16. http://www.ncbi.nlm.nih.gov/pubmed/17804020   full pdf available.

339   Stansbury, Jill, et al. "Promoting Healthy Thyroid Function with Iodine, Bladderwrack, Guggul and Iris." Journal of Restorative Medicine 1, no. 1 (2012): 83-90. doi:10.14200/jrm.2012.1.1008

340   Eaton, Jason R. "Mercury Poisoning & Pelotherapy Green Healing Clay (Bentonite, Montmorillonite, Illite)." *Mercury Poisoning, Mercury Toxicity and Green Healing Clays.* Eaton's Earth, 2014. Web. 19 Sept. 2016. <http://www.eytonsearth.org/mercury-toxicity-bentonite-clay.php>.

341   Fernández-Ruiz et al. "Cannabidiol for neurodegenerative disorders: important new clinical applications for this phytocannabinoid?" *British Journal of Clinical Pharmacology* 75, no. 2 (2013): 323-33. doi:10.1111/j.1365-2125.2012.04341.x.

342   Albert, Paul. "Vitamin D: The Alternative Hypothesis." Letter. 04 Aug. 2009. *Http://gettingstronger.org/.* Weill Cornell Medical College, 04 Aug. 2009. Web.

343   Waterhouse, Joyce C.. et al. "Reversing Bacteria-induced Vitamin D Receptor Dysfunction Is Key to Autoimmune Disease." *Annals of the New York Academy of Sciences* 1173.1 (2009): 757-65. Web. Sept. 2009. <http://www.ncbi.nlm.nih.gov/pubmed/19758226>.

344   Kivity, Shaye, Nancy Agmon-Levin, Michael Zisappl, and Yinon Shapira. "Vitamin D and Autoimmune Thyroid Diseases." *Cell Mol Immunol Cellular and Molecular Immunology* 8.3 (2011): 243-47. Web. Jan. 2011. <http://www.nature.com/cmi/journal/v8/n3/full/cmi201073a.html>.

345   Tainio, Bruce. "Vibrational Frequency List." *Just a List....:.* Blog, 13 Mar. 2008. Web. <http://justalist.blogspot.com/2008/03/vibrational-frequency-list.html>.